DON'T GUESS

Here's the calorie counter that has revolutionized dieting.

THE 1975 CALORIE GUIDE TO BRAND NAMES & BASIC FOODS is packed with thousands of foods you really eat, and takes the guesswork out of losing weight.

Now you can keep count while you fill your supermarket basket with the delicious favorites that will add up to a new slimmer you.

**THE BARBARA KRAUS
1975 CALORIE GUIDE
TO BRAND NAMES
AND BASIC FOODS**

SIGNET and PLUME Books of Interest

☐ **THE BARBARA KRAUS 1975 CARBOHYDRATE GUIDE TO BRAND NAMES AND BASIC FOODS by Barbara Kraus.** From the author of **Calories and Carbohydrates** comes a handy, portable, up-to-date carbohydrate counter that will let you keep track of your grams. It's a feast of information about thousands of foods for people who love to eat but need to know the carbohydrate count of their meals.
(#Y6661—$1.25)

☐ **CALORIES AND CARBOHYDRATES by Barbara Kraus.** Foreword by Edward B. Greenspan, M.D. This dictionary contains 7,500 brand names and basic foods with their caloric and carbohydrate counts. Recommended by doctors, nutritionists, and family food planners as an indispensable aid to those who must be concerned with what they eat, it will become the most important diet reference source you will ever own. (#J6441—$1.95)

☐ **THE DICTIONARY OF CALORIES AND CARBOHYDRATES by Barbara Kraus.** An ABC listing of over 9,000 brand names and basic foods with their caloric and carbohydrate count. The new, revised edition of **Calories and Carbohydrates**—the most complete and comprehensive guide in existence.
(#Z5079—$2.95)

☐ **SIX-WEEK MAKE YOURSELF OVER PLAN by Dolly Wageman.** Here is a unique, easy-to-follow and fun makeover program that has been developed by leading authorities in the field of exercise and weight control. (#Y5381—$1.25)

☐ **LET'S EAT RIGHT TO KEEP FIT by Adelle Davis.** Sensible, practical advice from America's foremost nutrition authority as to what vitamins, minerals and food balances you require, and the warning signs of diet deficiencies. (#J6336—$1.95)

THE NEW AMERICAN LIBRARY, INC.,
P.O. Box 999, Bergenfield, New Jersey 07621

Please send me the SIGNET and PLUME BOOKS I have checked above. I am enclosing $_____(check or money order—no currency or C.O.D.'s). Please include the list price plus 25¢ a copy to cover handling and mailing costs. (Prices and numbers are subject to change without notice.)

Name_____

Address_____

City_____State_____Zip Code_____
Allow at least 3 weeks for delivery

The Barbara Kraus 1975 Calorie Guide to Brand Names and Basic Foods

A SIGNET BOOK
NEW AMERICAN LIBRARY
TIMES MIRROR

*For Mon Ling,
Karl and Ling Ling Landegger*

COPYRIGHT © 1971, 1973, 1975 BY BARBARA KRAUS

All rights reserved

Excerpted from *Calories and Carbohydrates*
and *Dictionary of Calories and Carbohydrates*

SIGNET TRADEMARK REG. U.S. PAT. OFF. AND FOREIGN COUNTRIES
REGISTERED TRADEMARK—MARCA REGISTRADA
HECHO EN CHICAGO, U.S.A.

SIGNET, SIGNET CLASSICS, MENTOR, PLUME
AND MERIDIAN BOOKS
*are published by The New American Library, Inc.,
1301 Avenue of the Americas, New York
New York 10019*

FIRST PRINTING, MARCH, 1975

1 2 3 4 5 6 7 8 9

PRINTED IN THE UNITED STATES OF AMERICA

Foreword

The composition of the foods we eat is not static: it changes from time to time. In the case of *brand-name* products, manufacturers alter their recipes to reflect the availability of ingredients, advances in technology, or improvements in formulae. Each year new products appear on the market and some old ones are discontinued.

Similarly, information on *basic foods* such as meats, vegetables, and fruits may also change as a result of the development of better analytical methods, different growing conditions, or new marketing practices. These changes, however, are usually relatively small as compared with those in manufactured products.

Because a book on the caloric or nutritive values of foods must be kept up-to-date, this handy calorie counter will be revised each year to provide you with the most current and accurate estimates available. Generous use of this little book will help you and your family to select the right foods and the proper number of calories each member requires to gain, lose, or maintain healthy and attractive weight.

Good eating in 1975! For 1976, we'll pick up the new products, drop any has-beens, and make whatever other necessary changes.

BARBARA KRAUS

Why This Book?

Some of the data presented here can be found in more detail in my best-selling *Calories and Carbohydrates,* a dictionary of 7,500 brand names and basic foods. Complete as it is, it is meant to be used as a reference book at home or in the office and not to be squeezed into a suit jacket or evening bag—it's just too big.

Therefore, responding to the need for a portable calorie guide, and one which can reflect food changes often, I have written this smaller and more handy version. The selection of material and the additional new entries provide the reader with pertinent data on thousands of products that they would prepare at home to take to work, eat in a restaurant or luncheonette, nibble on from the coffee cart, take to the beach, buy in the candy store, etc.

For the sake of saving space and providing you with a greater selection of products, I had to make certain compromises: whereas in the giant book there are several physical descriptions of a product, here there is but one. When there is only one-calorie variance between brands, both products will bear the same number; such variances are not only unimportant in dieting, but they also are often due only to a different way of rounding numbers. Finally, no dietetic products are included that are dietetic only because they are sodium-restricted, as the calories are not affected.

For Beginners Only

The language of dieting is no more difficult to learn than any other new subject; in many respects, it's much easier, particularly if you restrict your education to clearly defined goals.

For you who never before had the need or the interest in a lesson in weight control, I offer the following elementary introduction, applicable to any diet, self-initiated or suggested by your doctor, nutritionist, or dietician.

A Calorie

An analysis of foods in terms of calories is most often the chosen method to describe the relative energy yielded by foods.

A calorie is a shorthand way to summarize the units of energy contained in any foodstuff or alcoholic beverage, similar to the way a thermometer indicates heat. One pound of fat is equal to 3,500 calories. Add this number of calories to those you need to balance your energy requirements and you will gain one pound; subtract it and you will lose a pound.

Other Nutrients

Carbohydrates—which include sugars, starches, and acids—are only one of several chemical compounds in foods that yield calories. Proteins, found mainly in beef, poultry, and fish; fats, found in oils, butter, marbling of meat, poultry skin; and alcohol, found in some beverages, also contribute calories. Except for alcohol, most foods contain at least some of all these nutrients.

The amount of carbohydrates varies from zero in meats and a trace in alcohol to a heavy concentration in sugar, syrups, some fruits, grains, and root vegetables.

As of this date, the most respected nutritional researchers insist that some carbohydrate is necessary every day for maintaining good health. The amount to be included is an individual matter, and in any drastic effort to change your eating patterns, be sure to consult your doctor first.

Now, on to how to use this new language.

To begin with, you use this book like a dictionary. If your plan is to cut down on calories, the easiest way to do so is to consult the portable calorie counter and keep an accurate count of your total intake of food and beverages for a period of seven days. If you have not gained or lost weight during that week, divide that number by seven and you'll have your maintenance diet expressed in calories. To lose weight, you must reduce your daily or weekly intake of calories below this maintenance level. (To gain, increase the intake.)

Keeping in mind that you want to stay healthy and eat well-balanced meals (which include the basic food groups: milk or milk products; meat, poultry, or fish; vegetables and fruits; and whole grain or enriched breads or cereals, as well as some fats or oils), you then start to cut down on your portions in order to reduce your intake of calories. There are many imaginative ways to diet without total withdrawal from one's favorite foods.

Once you know and don't have to guess what calories are in your foods, you can relax and enjoy it. It could turn out that dieting isn't so bad after all.

ABBREVIATIONS AND SYMBOLS

* = prepared as package directs[1]
< = less than
& = and
" = inch
canned = bottles or jars as well as cans
dia. = diameter
fl. = fluid
liq. = liquid
lb. = pound
med. = medium

oz = ounce
pkg. = package
pt. = pint
qt. = quart
sq. = square
T. = tablespoon
Tr. = trace
tsp. = teaspoon
wt. = weight

Italics or name in parentheses = registered trademark, ®. All data not identified by company or trademark are based on material obtained from the United States Department of Agriculture.

EQUIVALENTS

By Weight

1 pound = 16 ounces
1 ounce = 28.35 grams
3.52 ounces = 100 grams

By Volume

1 quart = 4 cups
1 cup = 8 fluid ounces
1 cup = ½ pint
1 cup = 16 tablespoons
2 tablespoons = 1 fluid ounce
1 tablespoon = 3 teaspoons
1 pound butter = 4 sticks or 2 cups

---

[1] If the package directions call for whole or skim milk, the data given here are for whole milk unless otherwise stated.

Food and Description	Measure or Quantity	Calories

A

Food and Description	Measure or Quantity	Calories
ALEXANDER COCKTAIL MIX (Holland House)	1 serving	69
ALMOND:		
In shell	½ cup	120
Shelled, plain (Blue Diamond)	½ cup	504
ANCHOVY, PICKLED	2 anchovies	4
***ANGEL FOOD CAKE MIX** (Pillsbury)	1/12 of cake	140
APPLE:		
Eaten with skin	2½" dia.	77
Eaten without skin	2½" dia.	68
APPLE BUTTER, CIDER (Smucker's)	1 T.	37
APPLE CIDER (Mott's)	8 fl. oz.	113
APPLE DRINK:		
(Hi-C)	8 fl. oz.	120
(Wagner)	8 fl. oz.	120
APPLE DUMPLING (Pepperidge Farm)	1 dumpling	276
APPLE FRITTER (Mrs. Paul's)	½ of 8-oz. pkg.	237
APPLE JACKS (Kellogg's)	1 cup	110
APPLE JELLY:		
Sweetened (Smucker's)	1 T.	49
Low calorie (Dia-Mel; Louis Sherry)	1 T.	6
Low calorie (Slenderella)	1 T.	25
Low calorie (Tillie Lewis)	1 T.	11
APPLE JUICE (Heinz)	5½-fl.-oz. can	88
APPLE PIE:		
(Drake's)	2-oz. pie	204
(McDonald's)	1 serving	269
Dutch (Mrs. Smith's)	⅛ of 8" pie	309
French (Hostess)	4½-oz. pie	447
Natural juice (Mrs. Smith's)	⅛ of 8" pie	340
APPLESAUCE:		
(Del Monte)	½ cup	119

Food and Description	Measure or Quantity	Calories
(Hunt's)	5-oz. can	94
Low calorie (Diet Delight)	½ cup	58
*APPLESAUCE CAKE MIX (Pillsbury)	1/12 of cake	200
APPLE TURNOVER (Pillsbury)	1 turnover	150
APRICOT:		
Fresh, whole	1 apricot	18
Canned, heavy syrup (Del Monte; Hunt's)	½ cup	103
Canned, unsweetened (Tillie Lewis)	½ of 8-oz. can	54
Dried (Del Monte)	¼ cup	77
APRICOT PRESERVE:		
Sweetened (Smucker's)	1 T.	49
Low calorie (Slenderella)	1 T.	28
APRICOT SOUR COCKTAIL, liquid mix (Holland House)	2 fl. oz.	86
AQUAVIT (Leroux)	1½ fl. oz.	112
ARTICHOKE, boiled	1 med. artichoke	125
ASPARAGUS:		
Boiled	1 spear (½" dia. at base)	3
Green:		
Spears & liq. (Green Giant)	1/3 of 15-oz. can	24
Spears & liq., *Le Sueur*	¼ of 1-lb. 3-oz. can	23
White:		
Spears (Del Monte)	½ cup	17
Spears, with butter sauce (Green Giant)	1/3 pkg.	45
*ASPARAGUS SOUP (Campbell)	1 cup	80
AUNT JEMIMA SYRUP	1 T.	53
AVOCADO:		
California	3⅛" avocado	369
Florida	3⅝" avocado	389
*AWAKE (Birds Eye)	¾ cup	82
AYDS	1 piece	26

B

BACO NOIR BURGUNDY (Great Western)	1 fl. oz.	26
BAC*OS (General Mills)	1 T.	29

Food and Description	Measure or Quantity	Calories
BACON, crisp, drained	1 med. slice	46
BACON BITS (McCormick)	1 T.	24
BACON, CANADIAN, drained	1-oz. cooked slice	79
BAGEL (Lender's):		
Egg	2-oz. bagel	164
Garlic, onion, poppyseed, rye	2-oz. bagel	161
Plain	2-oz. bagel	156
Raisin	2-oz. bagel	166
BAKING POWDER (Royal)	1 T.	15
BAKON DELITES (Wise):		
Regular	½-oz. bag	72
Barbecue flavor	½-oz. bag	70
BAMBOO SHOOTS, sliced (La Choy)	½ cup	6
BANANA, unpeeled (Dole)	7-inch banana	114
BANANA PIE, cream (Morton)	⅙ of 16-oz. pie	190
BANANA PUDDING (Del Monte)	5-oz. can	187
BARBECUE DINNER MIX (Hunt's)	¼ of 2-lb. pkg.	384
BARDOLINO WINE (Antinori)	1 fl. oz.	28
BASS:		
Baked, stuffed	3 oz.	220
Oven-fried	3 oz.	166
B & B LIQUEUR	1½ fl. oz.	141
BEAN, BAKED:		
(B & M)	½ cup	180
In molasses sauce (Heinz)	½ cup	142
& brown sugar sauce (Campbell)	½ cup	155
With pork (Hunt's-*Snack Pack*)	5-oz. can	169
With pork & molasses sauce (Heinz) Boston-style	½ cup	152
With pork & tomato sauce:		
(Campbell)	½ cup	131
(Heinz)	½ cup	146
(Libby's)	½ cup	143
(Morton House)	¼ of 1-lb. can	140
With tomato sauce:		
(Heinz-*Campside*)	½ cup	175
(Heinz) vegetarian	½ cup	134
(Van Camp)	½ cup	143
BEAN & FRANKFURTER:		
(Campbell)	½ cup	182

Food and Description	Measure or Quantity	Calories
(Heinz)	½ cup	200
(Van Camp-*Beanie-Weenee*)	½ cup	158
BEAN & FRANKFURTER DINNER:		
(Banquet)	10¾-oz. dinner	528
(Morton)	12-oz. dinner	547
BEAN, GREEN:		
Boiled, 1½" to 2" pieces, drained	½ cup	17
Drained (Comstock)	½ cup	13
Solids & liq. (Green Giant)	¼ of 1-lb. can	19
In butter sauce (Green Giant)	½ pkg.	51
In mushroom sauce (Green Giant)	½ pkg.	55
With onion & bacon (Green Giant)	½ pkg.	55
With sliced mushrooms (Birds Eye)	½ pkg.	54
With toasted almonds (Birds Eye)	½ cup	52
BEAN, KIDNEY with chili gravy (Nalley's)	4 oz.	120
BEAN, LIMA:		
Boiled, drained	½ cup	94
Baby (Birds Eye)	½ cup	111
In butter sauce (Green Giant)	½ pkg.	174
Fordhook (Birds Eye)	½ pkg.	141
BEAN, REFRIED (Gebhardt)	½ cup	120
BEAN SALAD:		
(Hunt's-*Snack Pack*)	5-oz. can	111
(Le Sueur)	¼ of 1-lb. can	86
BEAN SOUP:		
With bacon (Campbell)	1 cup	152
With smoked ham (Heinz-*Great American*)	1 cup	201
BEAN SOUP, BLACK:		
* (Campbell)	1 cup	91
(Crosse & Blackwell)	½ of 13-oz. can	96
BEAN SOUP MIX (Lipton-*Cup-a-Soup*)	1 pkg.	111
BEAN SPROUT, canned (Chun King)	½ cup	20
BEAN, YELLOW:		
Boiled, 1" pieces, drained	½ cup	18
Canned, drained (Butter Kernel)	½ cup	20
Cut (Birds Eye)	½ pkg.	36
BEAUJOLAIS WINE:		
(B & G) St. Louis	1 fl. oz.	20
(Chanson) St. Vincent	1 fl. oz.	26
(Cruse)	1 fl. oz.	24

Food and Description	Measure or Quantity	Calories
BEECHNUT, shelled	1 oz.	161
BEEF, choice grade, medium done:		
Brisket, braised:		
Lean & fat	3 oz.	350
Lean only	3 oz.	189
Chuck, pot-roasted:		
Lean & fat	3 oz.	278
Lean only	3 oz.	182
Fat, separable, cooked	1 oz.	207
Filet Mignon. See Steak, sirloin, lean		
Flank, braised, 100% lean	3 oz.	167
Ground:		
Regular, broiled	3 oz.	243
Lean:		
Raw	½ cup	203
Broiled	3 oz.	186
Rib:		
Roasted, lean & fat	3 oz.	374
Roasted, lean only	3 oz.	205
Round:		
Broiled, lean & fat	3 oz.	222
Broiled, lean only	3 oz.	161
Rump:		
Roasted, lean & fat	3 oz.	295
Roasted, lean only	3 oz.	177
Steak, club, broiled:		
One 8-oz. steak (weighed without bone before cooking) will give you:		
Lean & fat	5.9 oz.	754
Lean only	3.4 oz.	234
Steak, porterhouse, broiled:		
One 16-oz. steak (weighed with bone before cooking) will give you:		
Lean & fat	10.2 oz.	1339
Lean only	5.9 oz.	372
Steak, ribeye, broiled:		
One 10-oz. steak (weighed without bone before cooking) will give you:		
Lean & fat	7.3 oz.	911
Lean only	3.8 oz.	258
Steak, sirloin, double-bone, broiled:		
One 16-oz. steak (weighed with bone before cooking) will give you:		
Lean & fat	8.9 oz.	1028
Lean only	5.9 oz.	359

Food and Description	Measure or Quantity	Calories
One 12-oz. steak (weighed with bone before cooking) will give you:		
Lean & fat	6.6 oz.	767
Lean only	4.4 oz.	268
Steak, T-bone, broiled:		
One 16-oz. steak (weighed with bone before cooking) will give you:		
Lean & fat	9.8 oz.	1315
Lean only	5.5 oz.	348
BEEF BOUILLON (Wyler's)	1 cube	10
BEEF, CHIPPED:		
Canned, creamed (Swanson)	½ cup	96
Frozen, creamed (Banquet)	5-oz. bag	126
BEEF DINNER:		
(Banquet)	11-oz. dinner	312
(Swanson) 3-course	15-oz dinner	567
Beef steak & carrots (Weight Watchers)	10-oz. luncheon	412
Beef steak & cauliflower (Weight Watchers)	11-oz. luncheon	431
Chopped (Banquet)	11-oz. dinner	443
Chopped sirloin (Swanson)	10 oz. dinner	447
Chopped (Weight Watchers)	18-oz. dinner	665
Sliced (Morton)	11-oz. dinner	290
Sliced (Morton) 3-course	16-oz. dinner	636
BEEF GOULASH (Heinz)	8½-oz. can	253
BEEF HASH, ROAST:		
Canned (Hormel-*Mary Kitchen*)	7½ oz.	390
Frozen (Stouffer's)	11½-oz. pkg.	460
BEEF JERKY:		
(Beatrice Foods-*Cow-Boy Jo's*)	¼-oz. piece	24
(General Mills)	¼-oz. piece	25
(Lowrey's)	¼-oz. piece	21
BEEF PATTIES, frozen (Morton House):		
& Burgundy	4⅛-oz. serving	154
& Italian sauce	4⅙-oz. serving	171
& Mexican sauce	4⅙-oz. serving	157
BEEF PIE:		
(Banquet)	8-oz. pie	409
(Morton)	8-oz. pie	368
(Swanson)	8-oz. pie	434
BEEF PUFFS (Durkee)	1 piece	47

Food and Description	Measure or Quantity	Calories
BEEF SOUP:		
(Campbell-*Chunky*)	1 cup	185
Broth (College Inn)	1 cup	19
*Consommé (Campbell)	1 cup	33
Mix, broth (Lipton-*Cup-a-Broth*)	1 pkg.	19
Mix, noodle (Lipton-*Cup-a-Soup*)	1 pkg.	34
*Noodle (Manischewitz)	1 cup	64
With dumplings (Heinz-*Great American*)	1 cup	109
BEEF STEW:		
Home recipe, made with lean beef chuck	1 cup	218
(Armour Star)	1/3 of 24-oz. can	197
(B & M)	1 cup	152
(Dinty Moore)	8 oz.	190
(Heinz)	8½-oz. can	253
(Morton House)	1/3 of 24-oz. can	241
BEEF STEW SEASONING MIX (Durkee)	1 pkg.	99
BEEF STROGANOFF (Hormel)	½ of 1-lb. can	322
BEEF STROGANOFF MIX (Jeno's)	¼ of 40-oz. pkg.	482
BEER & ALE:		
Regular:		
Andeker	8 fl. oz.	110
Black Horse Ale, 5% alcohol	8 fl. oz.	108
Black Label, 4.9% alcohol	8 fl. oz.	93
Buckeye, 4.6% alcohol	8 fl. oz.	96
Budweiser, 4.9% alcohol	8 fl. oz.	104
Budweiser, 3.9% alcohol	8 fl. oz.	91
Busch, Bavarian, 4.9% alcohol	8 fl. oz.	104
Busch Bavarian, 3.9% alcohol	8 fl. oz.	91
Eastside Lager	8 fl. oz.	97
Hamm's	8 fl. oz.	101
Heidelberg, 4.6% alcohol	8 fl. oz.	89
Knickerbocker, 4.6% alcohol	8 fl. oz.	107
Meister Brau Premium, regular or draft, 4.6% alcohol	8 fl. oz.	96
Michelob, 4.9% alcohol	8 fl. oz.	107
Narrangansett, 4.7% alcohol	8 fl. oz.	103
North Star, regular	8 fl. oz.	110
North Star, 3.2 low gravity	8 fl. oz.	95
Pabst Blue Ribbon	8 fl. oz.	100
Pfeifer, regular	8 fl. oz.	110
Pfeifer, 3.2 low gravity	8 fl. oz.	95
Red Cap, 5.6% alcohol	8 fl. oz.	102
Rheingold, 4.6% alcohol	8 fl. oz.	107
Schlitz	8 fl. oz.	103
Schmidt, regular or extra special	8 fl. oz.	110

Food and Description	Measure or Quantity	Calories
Schmidt, 3.2 low gravity	8 fl. oz.	95
Stag, 4.8% alcohol	8 fl. oz.	91
Tuborg, USA, 4.8% alcohol	8 fl. oz.	93
Yuengling, premium	8 fl. oz.	96
Low carbohydrate:		
Dia-beer	8 fl. oz.	97
Gablinger's, 4.5% alcohol	8 fl. oz.	66
Meister Brau Lite, 4.6% alcohol	8 fl. oz.	64
BEER, NEAR:		
Kingsbury (Heileman) 0.4% alcohol	8 fl. oz.	41
(Metbrew) 0.4 % alcohol	8 fl. oz.	49
BEET:		
Boiled, whole	2″ dia. beet	16
Boiled, sliced	½ cup	33
Drained (Del Monte)	½ cup	26
Harvard, solids & liq. (Greenwood's)	½ cup	50
Pickled, drained (Greenwood's)	½ cup	40
Pickled with onion, drained (Greenwood's)	½ cup	45
BENEDICTINE LIQUEUR (Julius Wile)	1½ fl. oz.	168
BERNKASTELER (Deinhard)	1 fl. oz.	20
BERRY PIE (Hostess)	4½-oz. pie	421
BIG MAC (McDonald's)	1 hamburger	561
BIG WHEEL (Hostess)	1 cake	185
BISCUIT, buttermilk (Pillsbury)	1 biscuit	60
BISCUIT DOUGH:		
(Borden-*Buttered-Up*)	1 piece	90
Baking powder (Pillsbury-*1869*) Heat 'n Serve	1 piece	100
BI-SICLE (Popsicle Industries)	3 fl. oz.	116
BITTER LEMON, soft drink:		
(Canada Dry)	8 fl. oz.	117
(Schweppes)	8 fl. oz.	128
BITTER ORANGE, soft drink (Schweppes)	8 fl. oz.	122
BITTERS (Angostura)	1 tsp.	14
BLACKBERRY, fresh, hulled	½ cup	42
BLACKBERRY BRANDY (DeKuyper)	1½ fl. oz.	128

Food and Description	Measure or Quantity	Calories
BLACKBERRY JELLY, low calorie (Smucker's)	1 T.	4
BLACKBERRY LIQUEUR (DeKuyper)	1½ fl. oz.	112
BLACKBERRY PIE (Banquet)	4-oz. serving	301
BLACKBERRY PRESERVE (Smucker's)	1 T.	53
BLACKBERRY SOUR COCKTAIL MIX (Holland House)	1½ fl. oz.	75
BLACKBERRY WINE (Mogen David)	1 fl. oz.	45
BLACK-EYED PEAS (Birds Eye)	½ cup	92
BLACK RUSSIAN COCKTAIL MIX (Holland House)	1½- fl. oz.	138
BLINTZE (Aunt Leah's) cheese	1 blintze	70
BLOODY MARY MIX:		
Dry (Bar-Tender's)	1 serving	26
Dry (Holland House)	1 serving	56
Liquid (Sacramento)	½ cup	28
BLUEBERRY:		
Fresh	½ cup	45
(Birds Eye)	½ cup	114
BLUEBERRY PIE:		
(Banquet)	4-oz. serving	293
(Hostess)	4½-oz. pie	421
(Morton)	⅛ of 24-oz. pie	289
(Mrs. Smith's) natural juice	⅙ of 8" pie	347
BLUEBERRY PRESERVE (Smucker's)	1 T.	52
BLUEBERRY TURNOVER (Pillsbury)	1 turnover	150
BLUEFISH, fried	3½"x3"x½"-piece	308
BOCKWURST	1-oz. slice	75
BOLOGNA:		
With cereal	1-oz. slice	74
(Armour Star) all meat	1-oz. slice	99
(Oscar Mayer) all meat	1-oz. slice	89
(Eckrich) ring	1-oz. slice	94
(Vienna)	1-oz. slice	77
(Wilson)	1-oz. slice	87

Food and Description	Measure or Quantity	Calories
BORDEAUX WINE (Cruse)	1 fl. oz.	21
BORSCHT (Manischewitz)	½ cup	36
BOSCO (Best Foods)	1 T.	57
BOSTON CREAM PIE (Mrs. Smith's)	⅛ of 8" pie	329
BOYSENBERRY JELLY (Smucker's)	1 T.	50
BOYSENBERRY PIE (Morton)	⅙ of 20-oz. pie	249
BRAN BREAKFAST CEREAL:		
Plain:		
All-Bran (Kellogg's)	½ cup	64
Bran Buds (Kellogg's)	⅓ cup	73
40% bran flakes (Kellogg's)	¾ cup	70
40% bran flakes (Post)	⅔ cup	97
100% bran (Nabisco)	½ cup	97
Raisin bran flakes:		
(Kellogg's)	¾ cup	101
(Post) regular or cinnamon	½ cup	92
BRANDY, FLAVORED:		
Blackberry (Garnier; Hiram Walker)	1 fl. oz.	86
Coffee (Old Mr. Boston)	1 fl. oz.	74
BRATWURST (Oscar Mayer)	1 oz.	94
BRAUNSCHWEIGER:		
(Oscar Mayer)	1-oz. slice	107
(Wilson)	1-oz. slice	90
Beef (Eckrich)	1-oz. slice	71
BRAZIL NUT, shelled	½ cup	458
BREAD:		
Boston brown	3"x¾" slice	101
Cheese, party (Pepperidge Farm)	6-gram slice	18
Cracked wheat, honey (Wonder)	.8-oz. slice	61
Date-nut (Thomas')	1.1-oz. slice	94
Finn Crisp	1 piece	22
French (Wonder)	1-oz. slice	75
Glutogen Gluten (Thomas')	.5-oz. slice	35
Italian (Pepperidge Farm)	1" slice	88
Natural Health (Arnold)	.9-oz. slice	73
Oatmeal (Arnold)	.8-oz. slice	64
Panettone (Van de Kamp's)	1-oz. slice	90
Profile (Wonder)	.8-oz. slice	59
Protogen Protein (Thomas')	.7-oz. slice	46
Pumpernickel:		
(Arnold) Jewish	1.4-oz. slice	104
(Levy's)	1.1-oz. slice	70
(Pepperidge Farm) party	8-gram slice	20

Food and Description	Measure or Quantity	Calories
Raisin, cinnamon (Thomas')	.8-oz. slice	60
Raisin, orange (Arnold)	.9-oz. slice	76
Rite Diet (Thomas')	.7-oz slice	50
Roman Meal	.8-oz. slice	63
Rye:		
(Levy's)	1.1-oz. slice	70
(Wonder) *Beefsteak*	.8-oz. slice	59
Ry-King:		
Brown	.4-oz. piece	43
Golden	10-gram piece	33
Lite	8-gram piece	30
Seasoned	9-gram piece	39
Sprouted Wheat (Mannafood)	1-oz. slice	58
Vienna	.8-oz. slice	67
Wheat berry (Wonder)	.8-oz. slice	56
Wheat, golden (Wonder)	.8-oz. slice	60
Wheat germ (Pepperidge Farm)	.9-oz. slice	68
White:		
(Arnold) Melba thin	.5-oz. slice	43
(Pepperidge Farm) large loaf	1-oz. slice	75
(Pepperidge Farm) sliced	.9-oz. slice	74
(Wonder) 32 to 'loaf	¾-oz. slice	55
Brick Oven (Arnold)	.8-oz. slice	68
Whole Wheat:		
(Arnold) Melba thin	.6-oz. slice	44
Brick Oven (Arnold)	.8-oz. slice	65
(Pepperidge Farm)	.9-oz. slice	62
BREAD, CANNED:		
Banana nut (Dromedary)	½" slice	75
Brown, plain or raisin (B & M)	½" slice	83
Chocolate nut (Dromedary)	½" slice	86
Date & nut (Crosse & Blackwell)	½" slice	65
Orange nut (Dromedary)	½" slice	78
BREAD MIX:		
*Apricot nut (Pillsbury)	1/12 of loaf	180
*Blueberry (Pillsbury)	1/12 of loaf	150
*Cranberry (Pillsbury)	1/12 of loaf	170
BREAD PUDDING, with raisins	½ cup	248
BREAD STICK, cheese, onion or salt (Keebler)	2 pieces	20
***BREAD STUFFING MIX** (Uncle Ben's *Stuff 'n Such*, with added butter)	½ cup	191
BRIGHT & EARLY	8 fl. oz.	132
BROADBEAN, Italian bean: (Birds Eye)	½ pkg.	34

Food and Description	Measure or Quantity	Calories
In tomato sauce (Green Giant)	½ pkg.	75
BROCCOLI:		
Boiled, whole stalk	2 stalks	94
Boiled, ½" pieces	½ cup	20
& noodles in sour cream sauce (Green Giant)	½ pkg.	143
In butter sauce (Green Giant)	½ pkg.	72
In cheese sauce (Green Giant)	½ pkg.	89
In Hollandaise sauce (Birds Eye)	½ pkg.	150
BROTWURST (Oscar Mayer)	3-oz. link	275
BRUSSELS SPROUT:		
Boiled	3-4 sprouts	28
Au gratin (Green Giant)	½ pkg.	106
In butter sauce (Green Giant)	½ pkg.	86
BUBBLE UP, sweetened	8 fl. oz.	97
BUC WHEATS, cereal (General Mills)	1 cup	102
BUCKWHEAT, cracked (Pocono)	1 oz.	104
BULGUR, canned, seasoned	½ cup	123
BURGUNDY WINE:		
(Gallo) regular or hearty	1 fl. oz.	17
(Great Western)	1 fl. oz.	23
(Inglenook) Navalle	1 fl. oz.	21
(Italian Swiss Colony)	1 fl. oz.	20
(Louis M. Martini)	1 fl. oz.	30
(Taylor)	1 fl. oz.	24
BURGUNDY WINE, SPARKLING:		
(B & G)	1 fl. oz.	23
(Great Western)	1 fl. oz.	29
(Inglenook) Vintage	1 fl. oz.	20
(Petri)	1 fl. oz.	21
BUTTER:		
Regular	1 T. (⅛ stick)	100
Regular	1 pat (1¼"x1¼"x⅓")	72
Whipped	1 T. (⅛ stick)	64
Whipped	1¼"x1¼"x⅓"-pat	29
BUTTERNUT, shelled	1 oz.	178
BUTTERSCOTCH PIE, cream (Banquet)	4-oz. serving	299
BUTTERSCOTCH PUDDING:		
Chilled (Breakstone)	5-oz. container	252
Chilled (Sealtest)	5-oz. container	155
Canned (Del Monte)	5-oz. can	191
Canned (Hunt's)	5-oz. can	238

Food and Description	Measure or Quantity	Calories

C

Food and Description	Measure or Quantity	Calories
CABBAGE, red, sweet & sour (Greenwood's)	½ cup	77
CABBAGE, white, boiled	½ cup	17
CABBAGE ROLLS stuffed with beef (Holloway House)	1 roll	184
CABERNET SAUVIGNON (Inglenook)	1 fl. oz.	19
CAKE:		
Plain:		
Without icing	⅑ of 9″ sq.	313
With boiled white icing	⅑ of 9″ sq.	401
With chocolate icing	1/12 of 10″ layer	489
With uncooked white icing	1/12 of 10″ layer	488
White:		
Without icing	⅑ of 9″ sq.	322
With coconut icing	1/12 of 10″ layer	493
With uncooked white icing	1/12 of 10″ layer	499
Yellow:		
Without icing	⅑ of 9″ sq.	312
With caramel icing	1/12 of 10″ layer	481
With chocolate icing, 2-layer	1/12 of 9″ cake	365
CAKE ICING, fudge (Pillsbury)	1/12 pkg.	150
CAKE MIX:		
*White (Pillsbury)	1/12 of cake	200
*Yellow:		
(Betty Crocker; Duncan Hines)	1/12 of cake	202
Butter recipe (Betty Crocker)	1/12 of cake	278
Golden butter (Duncan Hines)	1/12 of cake	283
(Swans Down)	1/12 of cake	186
CAMPARI	1½ fl. oz.	99
CANDY (See also **CANDY, DIETETIC**):		
Air Bon (Whitman's)	1 piece	10
Almonds, chocolate-covered (Kraft)	1 piece	14
Almond cluster (Kraft)	1 piece	63
Almond cluster (Peter Paul)	1 3/16-oz. pkg.	171
Almond Joy (Peter Paul)	1 ¾-oz. pkg.	231
Baby Ruth (Curtiss)	1 oz.	135
Baffle Bar (Cardinet's)	1 ¾-oz. bar	189
Berries (Mason)	1 oz.	100
Butterfinger (Curtiss)	1 oz.	134
Butternut (Hollywood)	1¼-oz. bar	168

Food and Description	Measure or Quantity	Calories
Butterscotch Skimmers (Nabisco)	1 piece	25
Candy corn (Brach's)	1 piece	7
Caramel:		
Chocolate (Kraft)	1 piece	33
Milk Duds (Holloway)	1 oz.	111
Milk Maid (Brach's)	1 piece	34
Vanilla (Kraft)	1 piece	33
Caravelle (Peter Paul)	1½ oz. pkg.	190
Carmallo (Queen Anne)	1 piece	83
Charleston Chew	10¢ size	149
Cherry, chocolate-covered (Brach's; Nabisco)	1 piece	66
Cherry-A-Let (Hoffman)	1 piece	215
Chewees (Curtiss)	1 oz.	116
Chocolate bar:		
Milk (Hershey's)	1.4-oz. bar	218
Semisweet (Nestlé's)	1 oz.	141
Special dark (Hershey's)	1.4-oz. bar	214
With almonds (Hershey's)	1.3-oz. bar	205
With almonds (Nestlé's)	1 oz.	149
Chocolate Crisp Bar (Kraft)	1 oz.	132
Chocolate Crunch Bar (Nestlé's)	1 oz.	140
Choc-Shop (Hoffman)	1 piece	241
Chunky	1 oz.	131
Cluster, peanut, chocolate-covered:		
(Brach's)	1 piece	79
(Hoffman)	1 piece	204
Coconut:		
Bar (Curtiss)	1 oz.	126
Bar (Nabisco *Welch's*)	1 piece	132
Bon Bons (Brach's)	1 piece	70
Cream Egg (Hershey's)	1 oz.	142
Dots (Mason)	1 oz.	100
Fiddle Faddle	1½-oz. packet	177
5th Avenue Bar (Luden's)	10¢ size	129
Fruit Roll (Sahadi):		
All flavors except apricot	1 piece	195
Apricot	1 piece	192
Fruit n' Nut Bar (Nestlé's)	1 oz.	140
Fudge, nut, bars or squares (Nabisco)	1 piece	71
Fudgies, bar (Kraft)	1 piece	27
Good & Fruity	1 oz.	106
Good & Plenty	1 oz.	100
Hard candy:		
Butterscotch (Brach's) disks	1 piece	23
Lemon drops (Brach's)	1 piece	15
(Reed's)	1 piece	17
Sour balls (Brach's)	1 piece	22
Stix Pak (Jolly Rancher)	1 piece	18
Hershey-Ets, candy-coated	1.1-oz. pkg.	154
Hershey-Ets, candy-coated	1 piece	5

Food and Description	Measure or Quantity	Calories
Hollywood	1½-oz. bar	183
Jelly beans (Brach's)	1 piece	11
Jelly nougats (Brach's)	1 piece	43
Jelly rings (Nabisco-*Chuckles*)	1 piece	37
Jube Jels (Brach's)	1 piece	11
Jujubes (Heide)	1 oz.	93
Jujubes (Nabisco-*Chuckles*)	1 piece	13
Jujyfruits (Heide)	1 oz.	94
Kisses (Hershey's)	1 piece	26
Krackel Bar (Hershey's)	1.4-oz. bar	212
Krackel Bar (Hershey's)	1 miniature	38
Licorice:		
Diamond Drops (Heide)	1 oz.	94
Twist (American Licorice Co.):		
Black	1 piece	27
Red	1 piece	33
Life Savers, drop	1 piece	10
Mallo Cup (Boyer)	10¢ size	173
Malted Milk Balls (Brach's)	1 piece	9
Mars Almond Bar	1 oz.	130
Marshmallow:		
(Kraft) miniature	1 piece	2
(Kraft) regular	1 piece	23
Mary Jane (Miller)	1¢ size	31
Milk Shake (Hollywood)	1¼-oz. bar	148
Milky Way	1 oz.	120
Mint or peppermint:		
After dinner (Richardson):		
Jelly center	1 oz.	104
No jelly center	1 oz.	109
Chocolate-covered (Richardson)	1 oz.	106
Jamaica or *Liberty* Mints (Nabisco)	1 piece	24
Merri-mints (Delson)	1 piece	30
Junior mint pattie (Nabisco)	1 piece	10
Peppermint pattie (Nabisco)	1 piece	64
Thin (Delson)	1 piece	45
Mounds (Peter Paul)	1⁹⁄₁₀-oz. pkg.	236
M & M's, plain or peanut	1 oz.	140
Mr. Goodbar (Hershey's)	1.8-oz. bar	283
Mr. Goodbar (Hershey's)	1 miniature	39
Necco, Canada mints or Wintergreen	1 piece	13
Necco Wafers	1 piece	7
Nibs (Y & S)	1¾-oz. pkg.	179
$100,000 Bar (Nestlé's)	1 oz.	121
Orange slices (Brach's)	1 piece	55
Orange slices (Nabisco-*Chuckles*)	1 piece	29
Payday (Hollywood)	1¼-oz. bar	154
Peaks (Mason)	1 oz.	175
Peanut, chocolate-covered:		
(BB)	1 oz.	158

Food and Description	Measure or Quantity	Calories
(Kraft)	1 piece	12
(Nabisco)	1 piece	24
Peanut, French Burnt (Brach's)	1 piece	5
Peanut Brittle:		
(Bonomo)	1 oz.	132
(*Jumbo Peanut Block Bar*– Planters)	1 oz.	139
Peanut butter cup:		
(Boyer)	1¼-oz. pkg.	216
(Reese's)	¼-oz. cup	37
(Reese's) 2 to pkg.	1 piece	133
(Reese's) 1 to pkg.	1 piece	177
Peanut Butter Egg (Reese's)	1 oz.	133
Pom Poms (Nabsico)	1 piece	14
Raisin, chocolate-covered:		
(Brach's; Nabisco)	1 piece	4
(*Raisinets*–BB)	5¢ size	140
Rally	1.8-oz. bar	260
Rally	1.4-oz. bar	202
Red Hot Dollars (Heide)	1 oz.	94
Snickers	1 oz.	130
Spearmint leaves:		
(Brach's)	1 piece	23
(Nabisco-*Chuckles*)	1 piece	27
Sprigs (Hershey)	1 oz.	136
Stark Wafer Roll	1¼-oz. piece	132
Stars, chocolate (Kraft)	1 piece	13
Sugar Babies (Nabisco)	1 piece	6
Sugar Daddy (Nabisco):		
Caramel sucker	1 piece	121
Nugget	1 piece	48
Sugar Mama (Nabisco)	1 piece	101
Sugar Wafer (F & F)	1¼-oz. pkg.	180
Taffy:		
(Brach's)	1 piece	28
Salt water (Brach's)	1 piece	31
Turkish (Bonomo)	5¢ bar	115
3 Musketeers	1 oz.	120
Tootsie Roll	5¢ size	87
Tootsie Roll, pop	5¢ size	110
Tootsie Roll, pop-drop	1 piece	18
Triple Decker bar (Nestlé's)	1 oz.	148
Twizzlers (Y & S):		
Licorice	1¾-oz. pkg.	183
Strawberry bars	1 oz.	102
U-No Bar (Cardinet's)	⅞-oz. bar	161
(*Walnut Hill*–F & F)	1⅜-oz. bar	177
CANDY, DIETETIC:		
Chocolate bar, milk (Estee)	¾-oz. bar	128
Chocolates, assorted, *Slimtreats*	1 piece	13
Creams, peppermint (Estee)	1 piece	49

Food and Description	Measure or Quantity	Calories
Gum drop (Estee)	1 piece	3
Hard candy, assorted (Estee)	1 piece	11
Mint, any flavor	1 piece	4
Nut, chocolate-covered (Estee)	1 piece	47
CANTALOUPE, whole	5″ dia.	68
CAPERS (Crosse & Blackwell)	1 tsp.	2
CAP'N CRUNCH, vanilla (Quaker)	¾ cup	116
CAPPELLA WINE (Italian Swiss Colony)	1 oz.	21
***CARAMEL CAKE MIX** (Betty Crocker; Duncan Hines)	1/12 of cake	202
***CARAMEL PUDDING** (Royal)	½ cup	194
CARNATION INSTANT BREAKFAST:		
Regular	1 pkg.	128
Special Morning	1 pkg.	188
CARROT:		
Boiled, slices	½ cup	24
Canned, solids & liq., *Le Sueur*	⅓ of 15-oz. can	31
Canned, drained (Butter Kernel)	½ cup	29
Frozen:		
Nuggets in butter sauce (Green Giant)	⅓ pkg.	52
Sliced, honey-glazed (Green Giant)	⅓ pkg.	77
With brown sugar glaze (Birds Eye)	½ cup	87
CASABA MELON	½ average melon	92
CASHEW NUT:		
Roasted	5 large or 8 med.	60
Freshnut	1 oz.	169
Dry roasted (Planters)	1 oz.	171
Dry roasted (Skippy)	1 oz.	164
Oil roasted (Planters; Skippy)	1 oz.	178
CATSUP:		
(Bama; Smucker's; Stokeley-Van Camp)	1 T.	19
(Del Monte)	1 T.	20
(Heinz)	1 T.	16
(Hunt's)	1 T.	18
(Tillie Lewis) dietetic	1 T.	8
CAULIFLOWER:		
Raw or boiled buds	½ cup	14
Frozen, au gratin (Stouffer's)	⅓ pkg.	113

Food and Description	Measure or Quantity	Calories
Frozen, cut, in butter sauce (Green Giant)	1/3 pkg.	37
Frozen, Hungarian, with sour cream (Green Giant)	1/3 pkg.	70
Frozen, in cheese sauce (Green Giant)	1/3 pkg.	63
CAVIAR:		
Pressed	1 oz.	90
Whole eggs	1 T.	42
CELERIAC ROOT, pared	4 oz.	45
CELERY:		
1 large outer stalk	8" x 1½" at root end	7
1 small inner stalk	5" x ¾"	3
***CELERY SOUP**, cream of:		
(Campbell)	1 cup	75
(Heinz)	1 cup	101
CERVELAT:		
Dry	1 oz.	128
Soft	1 oz.	87
CHABLIS WINE:		
(B & G; Inglenook-Navalle)	1 fl. oz.	20
(Gallo)	1 fl. oz.	17
(Great Western)	1 fl. oz.	23
(Italian Swiss Colony) gold	1 fl. oz.	22
CHAMPAGNE:		
(Bollinger)	1 fl. oz.	24
(Gold Seal) pink, extra dry	1 fl. oz.	29
(Great Western):		
Regular	1 fl. oz.	28
Brut or Special Reserve	1 fl. oz.	25
Extra dry or pink	1 fl. oz.	26
(Lejon)	1 fl. oz.	22
(Mumm's) Cordon Rouge, brut	1 fl. oz.	22
(Mumm's) extra dry	1 fl. oz.	27
(Taylor) dry	1 fl. oz.	26
CHARLOTTE RUSSE, homemade	4 oz.	324
CHATEAUNEUF-DU-PAPE:		
(B & G)	1 fl. oz.	23
(Chanson)	1 fl. oz.	30
CHEERIOS	1¼ cups	112
CHEESE:		
American or cheddar:		
Natural:		
Cube	1" cube	68
(Kraft)	1 oz.	113

Food and Description	Measure or Quantity	Calories
Grated (Kraft)	1 oz.	129
Sharp cheddar, *Wispride*	1 T.	50
Process:		
(Borden)	¾-oz. slice	83
(Kraft)	1-oz. slice	106
(*Miracle Melt*–Borden):		
American	1 T.	38
Cheddar	1 T.	99
American Blue (Borden-*Miracle Melt*)	1 T.	38
Blue:		
(Foremost Blue Moon)	1 T.	52
Danish or Flora Donica (Borden)	1 oz.	105
Brick (Kraft) natural	1 oz.	103
Camembert, domestic (Borden; Kraft)	1 oz.	86
Caraway (Kraft) natural	1 oz.	111
Colby (Borden; Kraft)	1 oz.	111
Cottage:		
Creamed, partially (Meadow Gold)	1 cup	204
Creamed, unflavored:		
(Axelrod; Dean)	8-oz. container	218
Light n' Lively (Sealtest)	1 cup	155
Lite Line (Borden)	1 cup	189
Tangy or tiny curd (Breakstone)	8-oz. container	216
Creamed, flavored:		
Chive (Sealtest)	1 cup	211
Peach-pineapple (Sealtest)	1 cup	228
Pineapple (Sealtest)	1 cup	222
Spring Green Salad (Sealtest)	1 cup	208
Uncreamed:		
(Dean)	8-oz. container	191
Skim milk (Breakstone)	8-oz. container	182
Cream cheese:		
Plain, unwhipped:		
(Borden)	1 oz.	101
(Breakstone; Kraft-*Hostess*; Sealtest)	1 oz.	98
Neufchâtel (Borden)	1 oz.	74
(*Philadelphia*–Kraft)	1 oz.	104
(*Philadelphia*, imitation–Kraft)	1 oz.	52
Plain, whipped (Breakstone *Temp-Tee*)	1 T.	32
Flavored, unwhipped:		
Chive or olive-pimento (Kraft-*Hostess*)	1 oz.	84
Pimento or pineapple (Kraft-*Hostess*)	1 oz.	86
Flavored, whipped (Kraft):		
Blue	1 oz.	97
Chive	1 oz.	92
Salami	1 oz.	88

Food and Description	Measure or Quantity	Calories
Edam, natural (Kraft)	1 oz.	104
Farmer (Dean)	1 oz.	46
Gorgonzola (Foremost Blue Moon)	1 oz.	110
Gouda:		
(Borden-*Dutch Maid*)	1 oz.	86
Baby (Foremost Blue Moon)	1 oz.	120
Natural (Kraft)	1 oz.	107
Gruyère (Borden)	1 oz.	93
Gruyère (Kraft; Swiss Knight)	1 oz.	101
Kisses (Borden)	1 piece	19
Liederkranz (Borden)	1 oz.	86
Limburger (Borden-*Dutch Maid*)	1 oz.	97
Monterey Jack (Borden; Frigo; Kraft)	1 oz.	103
Mozzarella:		
(Borden)	1 oz.	96
Pizza, natural (Kraft)	1 oz.	79
Muenster:		
Natural (Borden)	1 oz.	85
Natural (Kraft)	1 oz.	100
Old English (Kraft)	1 oz.	105
Parmesan, grated:		
(Borden)	1 oz.	143
(Kraft)	1 oz.	127
Parmesan & Romano, grated:		
(Borden) natural	1 oz.	135
(Kraft)	1 oz.	130
Pimento American, process (Borden; Kraft)	1 oz.	104
Pizza:		
(Borden; Kraft)	1 oz.	85
(Frigo)	1 oz.	73
Port du Salut:		
(Foremost Blue Moon; Kraft)	1 oz.	100
Provolone:		
(Borden)	1 oz.	93
(Frigo; Kraft)	1 oz.	99
Ricotta:		
Moist (Borden)	1 oz.	42
(Sierra)	1 oz.	50
Romano, grated:		
(Borden)	1 oz.	136
(Buitoni)	1 oz.	123
Romano & Parmesan (Kraft)	1 oz.	133
Roquefort (Kraft)	1 oz.	105
Swiss, domestic:		
Natural (Borden; Foremost Blue Moon; Kraft)	1 oz.	104
Process (Borden):		
1-lb. pkg.	1 slice	64
6-oz. or 12-oz. pkg.	1 slice	72
½-lb. or 5-lb. pkg.	1 slice	78

Food and Description	Measure or Quantity	Calories
Swiss, Imported (Borden) Finland or Switzerland	1 oz.	104
CHEESE CAKE (Mrs. Smith's)	⅛ of 8" cake	306
CHEESE FONDUE (Borden)	6-oz. serving	354
CHEESE FOOD:		
(Borden)	1" x 1" x 1" piece	71
(Kraft)	1-oz. slice	93
Grated (Borden)	1 oz.	129
Grated, used in *Kraft Dinner*	1 oz.	129
Cheez 'n bacon, slices (Kraft)	¾-oz. slice	76
Pimento (Borden)	1 oz.	91
Pimento (Kraft)	1 oz. slice	94
Swiss:		
(Borden)	.7-oz. slice	68
(Borden)	.8-oz. slice	75
Cold-pack (Borden)	.7-oz. slice	62
Cold-pack (Borden)	.8-oz. slice	67
CHEESE PIE:		
(Tastykake)	4-oz. pie	357
Frozen, pineapple (Mrs. Smith's)	⅙ of 8" pie	273
CHEESE PUFF (Durkee)	1 piece	59
CHEESE SOUFFLÉ	¼ of 7" soufflé	240
CHEESE SPREAD:		
American or cheddar:		
(Borden)	.7-oz. slice	63
(Borden)	.8-oz. slice	69
(Nabisco-*Snack Mate*)	1 tsp.	15
Bacon (Borden) cheese 'n	1 oz.	72
Blue (Borden)	1 oz.	82
Cheddar, sharp (Borden-*Country Store*)	1 oz.	85
Cheez Whiz (Kraft)	1 oz.	76
Garlic (Borden)	1 oz.	72
Garlic (Kraft-*Squeeze-A-Snak*)	1 oz.	84
Hickory smoke (Nabisco-*Snack Mate*)	1 tsp.	14
Imitation (Kraft-*Tasty-loaf*)	1 oz.	48
Neufchâtel:		
Bacon & horseradish (Kraft-*Party Snack*)	1 oz.	74
Chipped beef, clam or pimento (Kraft-*Party Snack*)	1 oz.	67
Pineapple (Borden)	1 oz.	81
Onion (Nabisco)	1 tsp.	15
Pimento (Borden-*Country Store*)	1 T.	36
Pimento (Sealtest)	1 oz.	77
Pimento, *Velveeta*	1 oz.	84
Pineapple (Borden)	1 T.	36

Food and Description	Measure or Quantity	Calories
Smoke (Kraft-*Squeeze-A-Snak*)	1 oz.	83
Smokey (Borden)	1 oz.	72
Velveeta (Kraft)	1 oz.	84
CHEESE STRAW, frozen (Durkee)	1 piece	29
CHELOIS WINE (Great Western)	1 fl. oz.	24
CHENIN BLANC WINE (Inglenook)	1 fl. oz.	20
CHERI SWISSE (Park Avenue Imports)	1½ fl. oz.	135
CHERRY, sweet:		
Fresh, with stems	½ cup	41
Canned with pits, heavy syrup (Stokely-Van Camp)	½ cup	97
Canned, pitted, heavy syrup (Del Monte)	½ cup	92
Canned, dietetic pack:		
Light (Tillie Lewis)	½ of 8-oz. can	54
Royal Anne (S & W-*Nutradiet*)	14 whole cherries	47
CHERRY BRANDY (DeKuyper)	1½ fl. oz.	132
CHERRY CAKE, shortcake (Mrs. Smith's)	⅙ of 9″ cake	394
***CHERRY CAKE MIX:**		
(Duncan Hines)	1/12 of cake	193
Upside down (Betty Crocker)	⅑ of cake	282
CHERRY, CANDIED (Liberty)	1 oz.	93
CHERRY DRINK (Wagner)	8 fl. oz.	110
CHERRY HEERING (Hiram Walker)	1 fl. oz.	80
CHERRY JELLY:		
Sweetened (Smucker's)	1 T.	50
Low calorie (Slenderella)	1 T.	26
CHERRY LIQUEUR (DeKuyper)	1½ fl. oz.	112
CHERRY, MARASCHINO (Liberty)	1 average cherry	8
CHERRY PIE:		
(Drake's)	2-oz. pie	203
(Hostess)	4½-oz. pie	427
Cherry-apple (Tastykake)	4-oz. pie	373
Frozen (Morton)	⅙ of 24-oz. pie	342
Frozen (Mrs. Smith's)	⅙ of 8″ pie	309
Frozen (Mrs. Smith's) natural juice	⅙ of 8″ pie	344
Frozen, tart (Pepperidge Farm)	3-oz. pie tart	277

Food and Description	Measure or Quantity	Calories
CHERRY PIE FILLING		
(Wilderness)	⅛ of 21-oz. can	120
CHERRY PRESERVE:		
Sweetened (Smucker's)	1 T.	52
Low calorie (Dia-Mel; Louis Sherry)	1 T.	6
CHERRY & BLACK CHERRY SOFT DRINK:		
Sweetened:		
(Canada Dry)	8 fl. oz.	128
(Clicquot Club; Cott; Mission)	8 fl. oz.	125
(Dr. Brown's; Key Food, Nedicks; Waldbaum)	8 fl. oz.	108
(Fanta; Shasta; Yukon Club)	8 fl. oz.	113
(Hoffman)	8 fl. oz.	116
(Salute)	8 fl. oz.	110
High protein (Yoo-Hoo)	8 fl. oz.	133
Unsweetened or low calorie:		
(Clicquot Club; Cott; Dr. Brown's; Key Food; No-Cal; Yukon Club)	8 fl. oz.	3
(Shasta) black	8 fl. oz.	<1
CHERRY TURNOVER (Pillsbury)	1 turnover	150
CHESTNUT, fresh, shelled	1 oz.	55
CHEWING GUM:		
Sweetened:		
Bazooka, bubble	1¢ size	18
Beechies; Chicklets	1 piece	6
Beech-Nut; Cinnamint; Fruit Punch; Peppermint or sour lemon (Clark); sour (Warner-Lambert, Teaberry)	1 stick	10
Beemans; Black Jack; Clove; Juicy Fruit	1 stick	9
Chicklets, tiny size	5¢ pkg.	65
Dentyne	1 piece	4
Doublemint, Spearmint (Wrigley's)	1 stick	8
Unsweetened or dietetic:		
Bazooka, bubble	1 piece	16
Bubble (Estee)	1 piece	3
(Clark; *Care*Free*-Beech-Nut)	1 stick	7
(Estee)	1 stick	4
(Harvey's)	1 stick	4
Peppermint (Amurol)	1 stick	5
CHIANTI WINE:		
(Antinori) Classico, or 1955 or vintage	1 fl. oz.	29
Brolio Classico	1 fl. oz.	22

Food and Description	Measure or Quantity	Calories
(Gancia) Classico	1 fl. oz.	25
(Italian Swiss Colony)	1 fl. oz.	21
(Louis M. Martini)	1 fl. oz.	30
CHICKEN:		
Broiler, cooked, meat only	3 oz.	116
Fryer, fried, meat & skin	3 oz.	212
Fryer, fried meat only	3 oz.	178
Fryer, fried, a 2½-pound chicken (weighed with bone before cooking) will give you:		
Back	1 back	139
Breast	½ breast	154
Leg or drumstick	1 leg	87
Neck	1 neck	121
Rib	1 rib	42
Thigh	1 thigh	118
Wing	1 wing	78
Fried skin	1 oz.	119
Hen & cock:		
Stewed, meat & skin	3 oz.	269
Stewed, dark meat only	3 oz.	176
Stewed, light meat only	3 oz.	153
Stewed, diced	½ cup	139
Roaster, roasted, dark or light meat without skin	3 oz.	156
CHICKEN A LA KING:		
Home recipe	½ cup	233
Canned (Richardson & Robbins)	1 cup	272
CHICKEN, BONED, CANNED		
(Lyden Farms) solids & liq.	5-oz. jar	229
(Swanson) with broth	5-oz. can	223
CHICKEN BOUILLON:		
(Croyden House; Herb-Ox) instant	1 tsp. or 1 packet	12
(Herb-Ox; Steero; Wyler's)	1 cube or 1 tsp.	6
* (Knorr Swiss)	6 fl. oz.	13
(Maggi)	1 cube or tsp.	8
CHICKEN, CREAMED, frozen		
(Stouffer's)	½ of 11½-oz. pkg.	306
CHICKEN DINNER or LUNCHEON:		
Canned:		
Noodle (Heinz)	8½-oz. can	186
Noodle with vegetables (Lynden Farms)	½ of 15-oz. can	217
Frozen:		
Boneless chicken (Swanson-*Hungry Man*)	19-oz. dinner	746

Food and Description	Measure or Quantity	Calories
(Morton) 3-course	16-oz. dinner	699
Creole (WeightWatchers)	12-oz. luncheon	211
& noodles (Banquet)	12-oz. dinner	374
Fried (Banquet)	12-oz. dinner	530
Fried (Morton) 3-course	15½-oz. dinner	722
CHICKEN FRICASSEE:		
Canned (College Inn)	½ cup	117
Canned (Richardson & Robbins)	½ cup	128
CHICKEN, FRIED (Banquet)	½ chicken	960
CHICKEN GIBLETS, fryer, fried	1 heart, gizzard and liver	151
CHICKEN LIVER:		
Chopped (Mrs. Kornberg's)	1 oz.	43
Puff, frozen (Durkee)	½-oz. piece	48
CHICKEN & NOODLES, canned		
(College Inn)	5-oz. serving	170
CHICKEN PIE:		
(Banquet)	8-oz. pie	427
(Morton; Swanson)	8-oz. pie	445
CHICKEN PUFF (Durkee)	½-oz. piece	49
CHICKEN SOUP:		
(Campbell) *Chunky*	1 cup	155
Broth:		
* (Campbell)	1 cup	53
(College Inn)	1 cup	30
Cream of:		
* (Campbell)	1 cup	87
(Heinz-*Great American*)	1 cup	108
Gumbo:		
* (Campbell)	1 cup	55
Creole (Heinz-*Great American*)	1 cup	96
& Kasha (Manischewitz)	1 cup	41
*& Noodle:		
* (Campbell)	1 cup	62
* (Manischewitz)	1 cup	46
With dumplings (Heinz-*Great American*)	1 cup	89
*& Rice (Campbell)	1 cup	49
*Vegetable (Heinz)	1 cup	85
CHICKEN SOUP MIX:		
Cream of (Lipton-*Cup-a-Soup*)	1 pkg.	95
Cream of (Wyler's)	1 pkg.	93
& Noodle:		
(Lipton *Cup-a-Soup*)	1 pkg.	38
* (Lipton-*Giggle*)	1 cup	76

Food and Description	Measure or Quantity	Calories
Ring noodle (Lipton *Cup-a-Soup*)	1 pkg.	55
With meat (Lipton-*Cup-a-Soup*)	1 pkg.	42
*& Rice (Lipton)	1 cup	62
*Vegetable (Lipton)	1 cup	74
Vegetable (Lipton-*Cup-a-Soup*)	1 pkg.	10
CHICKEN SPREAD (Underwood)	1 tsp.	10
CHICKEN STEW:		
(B & M)	1 cup	128
(Swanson)	1 cup	166
With dumplings (Heinz)	8.5-oz. can	202
CHICKEN TAMALE PIE (Lynden Farms)	½ tamale pie	143
CHICORY, WITLOOF, cut	½ cup	4
CHILI OR CHILI CON CARNE:		
Canned with beans:		
(Chef Boy-Ar-Dee)	¼ of 30-oz. can	307
(Heinz)	8¾-oz. can	352
(Hormel)	7½ oz.	320
(Morton House)	1 cup	367
(Rosarita)	8 oz.	376
(Van Camp)	1 cup	304
Canned without beans:		
(Gebhardt)	8-oz. can	408
(Hormel)	7½ oz.	340
(Van Camp)	1 cup	460
CHILI SAUCE:		
(Del Monte; Heinz)	1 T.	18
(Hunt's)	1 T.	19
(Stokely-Van Camp)	1 T.	15
CHILI SEASONING MIX:		
(Durkee)	1 pkg.	148
*(Durkee)	1 cup	391
CHINESE DINNER:		
Beef chop suey (Chun King)	11 oz. dinner	310
Chicken chow mein (Banquet)	12-oz. dinner	282
Chicken chow mein (Chun King)	11-oz. dinner	350
Egg foo young (Chun King)	11-oz. dinner	340
Shrimp chow mein (Chun King)	11-oz. dinner	340
(Swanson)	11-oz. dinner	356
CHOCOLATE BAKING (Hershey's):		
Bitter	1 oz.	183
Semisweet chips	¼ cup	227
Sweetened chips, milk	¼ cup	234
CHOCOLATE CAKE, frozen:		
Fudge (Pepperidge Farm)	⅛ of cake	315
German (Sara Lee)	3 oz.	273

Food and Description	Measure or Quantity	Calories
German chocolate (Morton)	2.2-oz. serving	230
Golden (Pepperidge Farm)	1/8 of cake	320
CHOCOLATE CAKE MIX:		
*Chocolate malt (Betty Crocker)	1/12 of cake	200
*Deep chocolate (Duncan Hines)	1/12 of cake	201
*Double Dutch (Pillsbury)	1/12 of cake	210
*German (Swans Down)	1/12 of cake	187
*Streusel (Pillsbury)	1/12 of cake	340
CHOCOLATE DRINK (Borden)	9½-fl.-oz. can	232
CHOCOLATE DRINK MIX:		
Dutch, instant (Borden)	2 heaping tsps.	87
Quik (Nestlé's)	2 heaping tsps.	56
CHOCOLATE EXTRACT (Durkee)	1 tsp.	7
CHOCOLATE, HOT, home recipe	1 cup	238
CHOCOLATE ICE CREAM:		
(Borden) 9.5% fat	¼ pt.	126
(Prestige) French	¼ pt.	182
(Sealtest)	¼ pt.	136
CHOCOLATE PIE:		
Chiffon, home recipe	1/6 of 9" pie	459
Cream (Mrs. Smith's)	1/6 of 8" pie	247
Meringue (Mrs. Smith's)	1/8 of 10" pie	514
Nut (Tastykake)	4½-oz. pie	451
(Banquet)	2½-oz. serving	202
Tart (Pepperidge Farm)	3-oz. pie tart	306
CHOCOLATE PUDDING:		
Home recipe	½ cup	192
Chilled (Breakstone):		
Dark chocolate	5-oz. container	256
Light chocolate	5-oz. container	254
Canned:		
(Betty Crocker; Thank You)	½ cup	175
(Hunt's)	5-oz. can	239
(My-T-Fine-*Rich 'N Ready*)	5-oz. can	191
Dark (Sanna-*Swiss Miss*)	5-oz. container	165
Dark 'N Sweet (Royal-*Creamerino*)	5-oz. can	250
Light (Sanna-*Swiss Miss*)	5-oz. container	153
Fudge (Del Monte)	5-oz. can	198
Fudge (Hunt's)	5-oz. can	229
Fudge (My-T-Fine-*Rich 'N Ready*)	5-oz. can	186
Milk chocolate (Del Monte)	5-oz. can	202
Milk chocolate (Royal-*Creamerino*)	5-oz. can	244
CHOCOLATE PUDDING MIX:		
*Regular (Royal)	½ cup	196
*Instant (Royal)	½ cup	194

Food and Description	Measure or Quantity	Calories
CHOCOLATE SOFT DRINK:		
Sweetened:		
(Clicquot Club; Cott; Mission)	8 fl. oz.	122
(Hoffman-*Cocoa Cooler*)	8 fl. oz.	118
(Yoo Hoo) high protein	8 fl. oz.	133
Low calorie:		
(Cott; Mission)	8 fl. oz.	3
(Hoffman; Shasta)	8 fl. oz.	1
(No-Cal)	8 fl. oz.	4
CHOCOLATE SYRUP:		
Sweetened:		
(Hershey's)	1 T.	44
(Smucker's)	1 T.	51
Low calorie (Slim-ette)	1 T.	9
CHOCO-NUT SUNDAE CONE		
(Sealtest)	2½ fl. oz.	186
CHOP SUEY		
Canned:		
Chicken (Mow Sang)	20-oz. can	113
Pork (Mow Sang)	20-oz. can	167
Frozen (Banquet)	12-oz. dinner	282
Mix (Durkee)	1⅝-oz. pkg.	128
*Mix (Durkee)	1 cup	318
CHOW CHOW (Crosse & Blackwell)	1 T.	6
CHOW MEIN:		
Canned (Chun King-*Divider-Pak*):		
Beef	7-oz. serving	110
Chicken	7-oz. serving	100
Mushroom	1 cup	50
Pork	7-oz. serving	160
Shrimp	7-oz. serving	90
Frozen:		
Chicken with rice (Swanson)	8½-oz. pkg.	188
Vegetable (Temple)	1 cup	68
Mix (Durkee)	1⅝-oz. pkg.	128
*Mix (Durkee)	1 cup	318
CHUTNEY, *Major Grey's* (Crosse & Blackwell)	1 T.	53
CINNAMON WITH SUGAR (French's)	1 tsp.	15
CITRUS COOLER (Hi-C)	8 fl. oz.	12
CLAM:		
Raw, all kinds, meat only	4 med. clams	65
Canned:		
Chopped & minced, solids & liq. (Doxee)	4 oz.	59

Food and Description	Measure or Quantity	Calories
Chopped, meat only (Doxee)	4 oz.	111
Solids & liq. (Bumble Bee)	4½-oz. can	66
Frozen, breaded (Mrs. Paul's)	5-oz. pkg.	506
CLAM CAKE, thins (Mrs. Paul's)	2½-oz. piece	147
CLAM CHOWDER:		
Manhattan, canned:		
(Crosse & Blackwell)	½ can (6½-oz.)	61
(Snow)	8-oz.	85
New England, canned:		
(Crosse & Blackwell)	½ can (6½-oz.)	101
(Snow)	⅓ of 15-oz. can	87
New England, mix (Lipton-*Cup-a-Soup*)	1 pkg.	102
CLAM COCKTAIL (Sau-Sea)	4-oz. jar.	80
CLAM FRITTERS	2" x 1¾" fritter	124
CLAM JUICE:		
(Doxee)	8 oz.	43
(Snow)	8 oz.	31
CLAM SOUP MIX (Wyler's)	1 pkg.	112
CLAM STICK, breaded (Mrs. Paul's)	.8-oz. piece	46
CLARET WINE:		
(Gold Seal)	1 fl. oz.	27
(Inglenook) Navalle	1 fl. oz.	20
CLORETS, gum	1 piece	6
CLUB SODA SOFT DRINK, any brand, regular or dietetic	(any quantity)	0
COCKTAIL HOST MIX (Holland House)	1½ fl. oz.	70
COCOA, dry (Droste; Hershey's)	1 T.	22
COCOA KRISPIES, cereal	¾ cup	111
COCOA MIX:		
Hot (Hershey's)	1-oz. packet	116
* (Kraft)	1 cup	129
(Nestlé's-*EverReady*)	3 heaping tsps.	105
Instant:		
(Hershey's)	¾-oz. packet	84
Marshmallow, *Swiss Miss*	1 oz.	117
Rich chocolate (Carnation)	1-oz. pkg.	109
COCOA PUFFS, cereal	1 cup	109
COCONUT:		
Fresh, meat only	2" x 2" x ½ piece	156
Dried:		
Angel Flake (Baker's)	½ cup	178
Chocolate (Durkee)	½ cup	176

Food and Description	Measure or Quantity	Calories
Lemon, orange, or peppermint (Durkee)	½ cup	181
Premium shred (Baker's)	½ cup	210
COCONUT CAKE (Pepperidge Farm)	⅙ of cake	323
***COCONUT CAKE MIX** (Duncan Hines)	1/12 of cake	200
COCONUT PIE:		
Cream:		
(Tastykake)	4-oz. pie	467
(Morton)	⅙ of 16-oz. pie	206
(Mrs. Smith's)	⅙ of 8″ pie	233
Tart (Pepperidge Farm)	3-oz. pie tart	310
Custard:		
(Banquet)	5-oz. serving	294
(Morton)	⅙ of 22-oz. pie	224
(Mrs. Smith)	⅙ of 8″ pie	265
Meringue (Mrs. Smith's)	⅛ of 10″ pie	438
***COCONUT PUDDING MIX** (Royal)	½ cup	184
COCO WHEATS, cereal	3 T.	132
COD, broiled	3 oz.	144
COFFEE:		
Regular:		
* (*Max Pax;* Maxwell House; *Yuban)	¾ cup	2
(*Kava*–Borden)	1 tsp.	3
Instant:		
* (Maxwell House; Yuban)	¾ cup	4
Nescafé	1 slightly rounded tsp.	4
Decaffeinated:		
Decaf	1 tsp.	4
**Sanka,* regular	¾ cup	2
*Freeze-dried (*Maxim; Sanka*)	¾ cup	4
COFFEE BRANDY (DeKuyper)	1½ fl. oz.	138
COFFEE CAKE:		
(Drake's) junior	1 cake	126
(Drake's) large	11-oz. cake	1195
(Drake's) small	2-oz. pkg.	280
Almond danish (Pillsbury)	1 piece	140
Butterfly (Mrs. Smith's)	2¾-oz. piece	299
Cherry (Mrs. Smith's)	2¾-oz. piece	238
Cinnamon (Pillsbury)	2″ x 4″ piece	105
Cinnamon, iced (Pillsbury)	1 roll	115
Cinnamon twist (Pepperidge Farm)	⅙ of cake	156
Danish, apple (Morton)	13.5-oz. cake	1130

Food and Description	Measure or Quantity	Calories
Danish, apple (Sara Lee)	1 oz.	84
Danish, caramel (Pillsbury)	1 roll	155
Danish, pecan twist (Morton)	12-oz. cake	1369
Danish tray pack (Mrs. Smith's)	1¾-oz. piece	190
Melt-A-Way (Morton)	13-oz. cake	1511
Meltaway (Mrs. Smith's)	2¾-oz. piece	351
Pecan roll (Mrs. Smith's)	2¾-oz. piece	396
*COFFEE CAKE MIX (Aunt Jemima)	⅛ of cake	182
COFFEE LIQUEUR (DeKuyper)	1½ fl. oz.	140
COLA SOFT DRINK:		
Sweetened:		
(Canada Dry-*Jamaica*; Key Food-cherry)	8 fl. oz.	100
(Clicquot Club; Cott; Mission)	8 fl. oz.	110
Coca-Cola	8 fl. oz.	97
(Hoffman; Royal Crown; Waldbaum)	8 fl. oz.	108
(Key Food)	8 fl. oz.	102
(*Mr. Cola; Pepsi-Cola;* Royal Crown)	8 fl. oz.	104
(*RC* with a twist; Salute)	8 fl. oz.	98
(Shasta)	8 fl. oz.	101
Low calorie:		
(Canada Dry; *Diet Pepsi; Diet Rite;* No-Cal; Shasta; *RC Cola; Tab*)	8 fl. oz.	<1
(Clicquot Club; Cott; Mission)	8 fl. oz.	3
(Dr. Brown's; Hoffman; Yukon Club)	8 fl. oz.	1
COLD DUCK WINE (Great Western) pink	1 fl. oz.	31
COLESLAW, not drained, made with mayonnaise-type salad dressing	4 oz.	112
COLLARDS:		
Leaves, cooked	½ cup	31
Frozen, chopped (Birds Eye)	⅓ pkg.	29
CONCENTRATE, cereal	⅓ cup	107
CONCORD WINE:		
(Gold Seal)	1 fl. oz.	42
(Mogen David)	1 fl. oz.	40
Red (Pleasant Valley)	1 fl. oz.	30
CONSOMME MADRILENE (Crosse & Blackwell)	½ of 13-oz. can	33
COOKIE:		
Almond crescent (Nabisco)	1 piece	34

Food and Description	Measure or Quantity	Calories
Almond toast (Stella D'oro)	1 piece	49
Angelica Goodies (Stella D'oro)	1 piece	100
Anginetti (Stella D'oro)	1 piece	28
Animal Cracker:		
(Nabisco-*Barnum's*)	1 piece	12
(Sunshine) regular	1 piece	10
(Sunshine) iced	1 piece	26
Anisette (Stella D'oro)	1 piece	39
Applesauce (Sunshine)	1 piece	86
Arrowroot (Sunshine)	1 piece	16
Assortment:		
(Stella D'oro-*Lady Stella*)	1 piece	37
(Sunshine-*Lady Joan*)	1 piece	42
(Sunshine-*Lady Joan*), iced	1 piece	47
Aunt Sally, iced (Sunshine)	1 piece	96
Bana-Bee (Nab)	1 piece	42
Big Treat (Sunshine)	1 piece	153
Bordeaux (Pepperidge Farm)	1 piece	36
Breakfast Treats (Stella D'oro)	1 piece	99
Brown edge wafers (Nabisco)	1 piece	28
Brownie:		
(Drake's) Junior	2/3-oz. cake	80
(Hostess) 2 to pkg.	1 piece	100
(Tastykake)	1 pkg.	242
Nut (Pepperidge Farm)	1 piece	54
Peanut butter (Tastykake)	1 pkg.	239
Pecan fudge (Keebler)	1 piece	115
Brussels (Pepperidge Farm)	1 piece	42
Butter (Nabisco; Sunshine)	1 piece	23
Buttercup (Keebler)	1 piece	24
Butterscotch Fudgies (Tastykake)	1 pkg.	251
Capri (Pepperidge Farm)	1 piece	82
Cardiff (Pepperidge Farm)	1 piece	18
Cherry Coolers (Sunshine)	1 piece	29
Chinese almond (Stella D'oro)	1 piece	178
Chocolate & chocolate-covered:		
Como (Stella D'oro)	1 piece	155
Creme (Wise)	1 piece	32
Peanut bars (Nabisco-*Ideal*)	1 piece	94
Pinwheels (Nabisco)	1 piece	139
Snaps (Nabisco)	1 piece	18
Snaps (Sunshine)	1 piece	14
Wafers (Nabisco-*Famous*)	1 piece	28
Chocolate chip:		
(Drake's)	1 piece	74
(Keebler) old fashioned	1 piece	80
(Nabisco)	1 piece	33
(Nabisco-*Chips Ahoy*)	1 piece	51
(Nabisco-*Family Favorites*)	1 piece	33
(Nabisco) snaps	1 piece	21
(Pepperidge Farm)	1 piece	52
(Sunshine-*Chip-A-Roos*)	1 piece	63

Food and Description	Measure or Quantity	Calories
(Tastykake-*Choc-O-Chip*)	1 piece	57
Cinnamon:		
Crisp (Keebler)	1 piece	17
Spice, vanilla sandwich (Nabisco-*Crinkles*)	1 piece	38
Sugar (Pepperidge Farm)	1 piece	52
Toast (Sunshine)	1 piece	13
Coconut:		
Bar (Nabisco)	1 piece	45
Bar (Sunshine)	1 piece	47
(Nabisco-*Family Favorites*)	1 piece	16
Chocolate chip (Nabisco)	1 piece	77
Chocolate chip (Sunshine)	1 piece	80
Chocolate drop (Keebler)	1 piece	75
(*Coconut Kiss*-Tastykake)	1 piece	80
(*Jumble* Drake's)	1 piece	52
(*Commodore* Keebler)	1 piece	65
(*Como Delight*-Stella D'oro)	1 piece	153
(*Cowboys and Indians*-Nabisco)	1 piece	10
Cream Lunch (Sunshine)	1 piece	45
Creme Wafer Stick (Dutch Twin)	1 piece	36
Creme Wafer Stick (Nabisco)	1 piece	50
Cup Custard (Sunshine)	1 piece	71
Devil's Food Cake (Nab)	1¼-oz. pkg.	135
Devil's Food Cake (Nabisco)	1 piece	49
Dixie Vanilla (Sunshine)	1 piece	60
Dresden (Pepperidge Farm)	1 piece	83
Egg Jumbo (Stella D'oro)	1 piece	40
Fig bar:		
(Keebler)	1 piece	71
(Nab-*Fig Newtons*)	1 piece	104
(Nabisco-*Fig Newtons*)	1 piece	57
(Sunshine)	1 piece	45
Fortune (Chun King)	1 piece	31
Fruit, iced (Nabisco)	1 piece	71
Fudge:		
(Sunshine)	1 piece	72
Chips (Pepperidge Farm)	1 piece	51
(*Fudge Stripes*-Keebler)	1 piece	57
Gingersnap:		
(Keebler)	1 piece	24
(Nabisco) old fashion	1 piece	29
(Sunshine)	1 piece	24
(*Zu Zu*-Nabisco)	1 piece	16
Golden Bars (Stella D'oro)	1 piece	123
Golden Fruit (Sunshine)	1 piece	61
Hermit bar, frosted (Tastykake)	1 pkg.	321
(*Home Plate*-Keebler)	1 piece	58
(*Hostest With The Mostest*-Stella D'oro)	1 piece	39
(*Hydox*-Sunshine):		
Regular or mint	1 piece	48

Food and Description	Measure or Quantity	Calories
Vanilla	1 piece	50
(*Jan Hagel*–Keebler)	1 piece	44
(*Keebies*–Keebler)	1 piece	51
Ladyfinger	3¼" x 1⅜" x 1⅛"	40
Lemon:		
(Sunshine)	1 piece	76
Jumble rings (Nabisco)	1 piece	68
(*Lemon Coolers*–Sunshine)	1 piece	29
Nut crunch (Pepperidge Farm)	1 piece	57
Snaps (Nabisco)	1 piece	17
(*Lido*–Pepperidge Farm)	1 piece	91
(*Lisbon*–Pepperidge Farm)	1 piece	28
Macaroon:		
Almond (Tastykake)	1 piece	168
Coconut (Nabisco–*Bake Shop*)	1 piece	87
Sandwich (Nabisco)	1 piece	71
(*Margherite*–Stella D'oro)	1 piece	73
(*Marquisette*–Pepperidge Farm)	1 piece	45
Marshmallow:		
(*Fancy Crests*–Nabisco)	1 piece	53
(Mallowmars–Nabisco)	1 piece	60
(*Mallow Puff*–Sunshine)	1 piece	63
(*Minarets*–Nabisco)	1 piece	46
Puffs (Nabisco)	1 piece	94
Sandwich (Nabisco)	1 piece	32
(*Twirls*–Nabisco)	1 piece	133
(*Milano*–Pepperidge Farm)	1 piece	62
(*Milano*, mint–Pepperidge Farm)	1 piece	76
Mint sandwich (Nabisco-*Mystic*)	1 piece	88
Molasses & Spice (Sunshine)	1 piece	67
(*Naples*–Pepperidge Farm)	1 piece	33
(*Nassau*–Pepperidge Farm)	1 piece	83
Oatmeal:		
(Drake's)	1 piece	69
(Keebler) old fashioned	1 piece	79
(Nabisco)	1 piece	82
(Nabisco-*Family Favorites*)	1 piece	24
(Sunshine)	1 piece	58
Iced (Sunshine)	1 piece	69
Irish (Pepperidge Farm)	1 piece	50
Peanut butter (Sunshine)	1 piece	79
Raisin (Nabisco-*Bake Shop*)	1 piece	77
Raisin (Pepperidge Farm)	1 piece	55
Raisin bar (Tastykake)	1 pkg.	298
Whole wheat (Drake's)	1 piece	75
(*Old Country Treats*–Stella D'oro)	1 piece	64
(*Orleans*–Pepperidge Farm)	1 piece	30
Peach-apricot pastry (Stella D'oro)	1 piece	99
Peanut & peanut butter:		
Bars, cocoa-covered		
(Nabisco-*Crowns*)	1 piece	92
Caramel logs (Nabisco-*Heydays*)	1 piece	122

Food and Description	Measure or Quantity	Calories
Creme patties (Nab)	1-oz. pkg.	148
Creme patties (Nabisco)	1 piece	34
Creme patties, cocoa-covered (Nabisco-*Fancy*)	1 piece	60
Patties (Sunshine)	1 piece	33
Sandwich (Nabisco-*Nutter Butter*)	1 piece	69
Pecan Sandies (Keebler)	1 piece	85
Penguins (Keebler)	1 piece	111
Pfefferneuse, spice drop Stella D'oro	1 piece	40
(*Pirouette*–Pepperidge Farm)	1 piece	38
(*Pitter Patter*–Keebler)	1 piece	84
(*Pizzelle Carolines*–Stella D'oro)	1 piece	49
Raisin, fruit biscuit (Nabisco)	1 piece	58
(*Rich'n Chips*–Keebler)	1 piece	73
(*Rochelle*–Pepperidge Farm)	1 piece	81
Sandwich, creme:		
(*Cameo*–Nabisco)	1 piece	68
Chocolate chip (Nabisco)	1 piece	73
Chocolate fudge:		
(Keebler)	1 piece	99
Assorted (Nabisco-*Cookie Break*)	1 piece	52
Chocolate (Nabisco-*Cookie Break*)	1 piece	53
(*Obit*–Sunshine)	1 piece	51
(*Oreo*–Nab) 4 to pkg.	1 piece	35
(*Oreo*–Nabisco)	1 piece	51
(*Oreo & Swiss*–Nab) 2¼ oz. pkg.	1 piece	53
(*Oreo & Swiss*, assortment–Nabisco)	1 piece	51
(*Pride*–Nabisco)	1 piece	55
(*Social Tea*–Nabisco)	1 piece	51
(*Swiss*–Nab) 1-oz. pkg.	1 piece	36
(Tom Houston)	1 piece	74
Vanilla (Keebler)	1 piece	82
Vanilla (Nabisco)	1 piece	52
Vienna Finger (Sunshine)	1 piece	71
Sesame (*Regina*–Stella D'oro)	1 piece	51
Shortbread or shortcake:		
(Nabisco-*Dandy*)	1 piece	46
(Pepperidge Farm)	1 piece	72
(*Lorna Doone*–Nab) 1-oz. pkg.	1 piece	34
(*Lorna Doone* (Nabisco)	1 piece	37
Pecan (Nabisco)	1 piece	80
(*Scotties*–Sunshine)	1 piece	39
Striped (Nabisco)	1 piece	50
Vanilla (Tastykake)	1 piece	59
(*Social Tea Biscuit*–Nabisco)	1 piece	21
Spiced wafers (Nabisco)	1 piece	41
(*Sprinkles*–Sunshine)	1 piece	57
Sugar cookie:		
(Keebler) old fashioned	1 piece	78
(Pepperidge Farm)	1 piece	51

Food and Description	Measure or Quantity	Calories
(Sunshine)	1 piece	86
Brown (Nabisco-*Family Favorite*)	1 piece	25
Brown (Pepperidge Farm)	1 piece	48
Rings (Nabisco)	1 piece	69
Sugar wafer:		
(Nab-*Biscos*; Sunshine)	1 piece	43
(Nabisco-*Biscos*)	1 piece	19
Assorted (Dutch Twin)	1 piece	34
Krisp Kreem (Keebler)	1 piece	31
Lemon (Sunshine)	1 piece	44
(*Swedish Kreme*-Keebler)	1 piece	98
(*Tahiti*-Pepperidge Farm)	1 piece	84
Toy (Sunshine)	1 piece	13
Vanilla creme (Wise)	1 piece	33
Vanilla snap (Nabisco)	1 piece	13
Vanilla wafer:		
(Keebler;Nabisco-*Nilla*)	1 piece	19
(Sunshine) small	1 piece	15
(*Venice*-Pepperidge Farm)	1 piece	57
Waffle creme (Dutch Twin)	1 piece	44
Waffle creme (Nabisco-*Biscos*)	1 piece	42
(*Yum Yums*-Sunshine)	1 piece	83
COOKIE, DIETETIC:		
Angel puffs (Stella D'oro)	1 piece	17
Apple pastry (Stella D'oro)	1 piece	94
Assorted wafers (Estee)	1 piece	26
Choco chip (Dia-Mel)	1 piece	40
Chocolate chip (Estee)	1 piece	32
Chocolate wafer (Estee)	1 piece	27
Fig pastry (Stella D'oro)	1 piece	100
Fruit wafer (Estee)	1 piece	27
Have-A-Heart (Stella D'oro)	1 piece	97
Holland bittersweet or milk wafer (Estee)	1 piece	127
Kichel (Stella D'oro)	1 piece	8
Oatmeal raisin (Estee)	1 piece	34
Peach-apricot pastry (Stella D'oro)	1 piece	104
Prune pastry (Stella D'oro)	1 piece	92
Royal Nuggets (Stella D'oro)	1 piece	2
Sandwich (Estee)	1 piece	55
Sandwich, lemon (Estee)	1 piece	57
Vanilla wafer (Estee)	1 piece	28
COOKIE DOUGH:		
Chocolate (Pillsbury)	1 cookie	53
Peanut butter (Pillsbury)	1 cookie	50
COOKIE MIX:		
Brownie:		
*Butterscotch (Betty Crocker)	1½" sq.	59
*"Cake like" (Duncan Hines)	1/24 of pan	148
*Fudge (Pillsbury)	1½" sq.	60

Food and Description	Measure or Quantity	Calories
*Fudge, chewy (Duncan Hines)	1/24 of pan	142
*German chocolate (Betty Crocker)	1½" sq.	70
*Walnut (Pillsbury)	1½" sq.	65
*Toll House, with morsels, prepared with egg (Nestlé's)	1 piece	52
COOL 'N CREAMY (Birds Eye)	½ cup	172
CORN:		
Fresh, boiled	5" x 1¾" ear	70
Canned, regular:		
Drained solids (Del Monte)	½ cup	78
Shoe Peg, *Le Sueur*	¼ of 17-oz. can	79
Solids & liq. (Green Giant)	½ of 8.5-oz. can	80
Solids & liq. (Stokely-Van Camp)	½ cup	74
Vacuum pack, white (Green Giant)	⅓ of 12-oz. can	100
Vacuum pack, yellow, *Niblets*	⅓ of 12-oz. can	95
With peppers, *Mexicorn*	⅓ of 12-oz. can	95
Canned, cream style:		
(Green Giant)	½ of 8.5-oz. can	107
(Stokely-Van Camp)	½ cup	94
Frozen:		
On the cob (Birds Eye)	1 ear	98
On the cob, *Niblet Ears*	1 ear	167
Kernel (Birds Eye)	½ cup	77
Cream style (Green Giant)	⅓ pkg.	74
In butter sauce, white (Green Giant)	⅓ pkg.	112
In butter sauce, yellow (Green Giant)	½ pkg.	90
CORNBREAD (Pillsbury)	1 piece	95
CORNBREAD MIX:		
(Albers)	1 oz.	109
*(Aunt Jemima)	⅙ of cornbread	226
*(Dromedary)	2" x 2" piece	125
*(Pillsbury-*Ballard*)	⅛ of recipe	160
CORN CHEX, cereal	1¼ cups	111
CORNED BEEF:		
Cooked, boneless, medium fat	3 oz.	316
Canned:		
(Armour Star)	¼ of 12-oz. can	242
(Hormel) *Dinty Moore*	3 oz.	190
Brisket (Wilson) *Tender Made*	3 oz.	135
Packaged:		
(Oscar Mayer)	5-gram slice	7
(Vienna)	1 oz.	68
CORNED BEEF HASH:		
(Austex)	⅕ of 15-oz. can	256

Food and Description	Measure or Quantity	Calories
(Libby's)	3 oz.	144
(Libby's) home-style	3 oz.	170
CORNED BEEF HASH DINNER		
(Banquet)	10-oz. dinner	372
CORNED BEEF SPREAD		
(Underwood)	1 tsp.	9
CORN FLAKES, cereal:		
Country (General Mills)	1¼ cups	111
(Kellogg's; Van Brode)	1 oz.	106
(Ralston Purina)	1 cup	109
CORN FRITTER (Mrs. Paul's)	½ of 8-oz. pkg.	281
CORN MEAL:		
Bolted (Aunt Jemima)	¼ cup	148
Degermed (Albers)	1 T.	36
CORN SOUFFLÉ (Stouffer's)	½ of 12-oz. pkg.	246
CORNSTARCH (Argo; Kingsford's; Duryea's)	1 tsp.	11
CORN SYRUP	1 T.	61
CORN TOTAL (General Mills)	1¼ cups	111
COUGH DROP:		
(Beech-Nut; Pine Bros.)	1 drop	10
(H-B; Luden's; Smith Bros.)	1 drop	8
(Estee)	1 drop	12
CRAB:		
Fresh:		
Steamed, whole	½ lb.	101
Steamed, meat only	½ cup	58
Canned:		
Alaska King (Del Monte)	½ of 7½-oz. can	101
King Crab (Icy Point; Pillar Rock)	½ of 7½-oz. can	108
Frozen (Wakefield's Alaska King)	4 oz.	46
CRAB APPLE JELLY (Smuckers)	1 T.	49
CRAB CAKE, thins (Mrs. Paul's)	2½-oz. cake	158
CRAB COCKTAIL (Sau-Sea)	4-oz. jar.	80
CRAB, DEVILED (Mrs. Paul's)	3-oz. crab	173
CRAB IMPERIAL, home recipe	½ cup	162
CRAB NEWBURG (Stouffer's)	½ of 12-oz. pkg.	281
CRAB SOUP (Crosse & Blackwell)	½ of 13-oz. can	59

Food and Description	Measure or Quantity	Calories
CRACKERS, PUFFS & CHIPS:		
American Harvest (Nabisco)	1 piece	16
Arrowroot biscuit (Nabisco)	1 piece	22
Bacon-flavored thins (Nabisco)	1 piece	11
Bacon Nips	1 oz.	147
Bacon rinds (Wonder)	1 oz.	146
Bacon toast (Keebler)	1 piece	15
(*Bacon Tasters*–Old London)	½-oz. bag	62
(*Bugles*–General Mills)	15 pieces	81
Butter thins (Nabisco)	1 piece	15
Cheese flavored:		
Cheese 'N Bacon, sandwich (Nab)	1 piece	30
Cheese'n cracker (Kraft)	4 crackers & ¾ oz. cheese	138
(*Cheese Nips*–Nabisco)	1 piece	5
Cheese on Rye, sandwich (Nab)	1 piece	32
(*Cheese Pixies*—Wise)	1-oz. bag.	163
Chee.Tos, fried or puffs	1 oz.	156
(*Cheeze Doodles*–Old London)	½-oz. pkg.	78
(*Cheez-Its*–Sunshine)	1 piece	6
(*Cheez Waffles*–Austin's)	1 piece	26
(*Cheez Waffles*–Old London)	1 piece	11
(*Che-zo*–Keebler)	1 piece	5
(*Combo Cheez*–Austin's)	1 piece	26
(*Ritz*–Nabisco)	1 piece	17
Sandwich (Nab)	1 piece	31
(*Shapies*, dip delights–Nabisco)	1 piece	9
Thins (Pepperidge Farms)	1 piece	12
Thins, dietetic (Estee)	1 piece	5
(*Tid-Bits*–Nabisco)	1 piece	4
Toast (Keebler)	1 piece	16
Twists (Nalley; Wonder)	1 oz.	155
Cheese & peanut butter sandwich:		
(Austin's)	1⅜-oz. pkg.	194
(*O-So-Gud*–Nab or variety pack)	1 piece	35
(*Chicken in a Biskit*–Nabisco)	1 piece	10
(*Chippers*–Nabisco)	1 piece	14
(*Chipsters*–Nabisco)	1 piece	2
Clam flavored crisps (Snow)	1 oz.	147
Club (Keebler)	1 piece	15
(*Corn Capers*–Wonder)	1 oz.	158
(*Corn Cheeze* (Tom Houston)	1 piece	3
Corn chips:		
Cornetts	1 oz.	153
Fritos	1 oz.	159
Fritos, barbecue	1 oz.	156
(*Korkers*–Nabisco)	1 piece	8
(Old London)	1-oz. bag	162
(Wise) rippled	1-oz. bag	162
(Wonder)	1 oz.	162
Barbecue (Wise)	1¾-oz. bag	274
(*Corn Diggers*–Nabisco)	1 piece	4

Food and Description	Measure or Quantity	Calories
(*Crown Pilot*—Nabisco)	1 piece	73
(*Dipsy Doodles*—Old London)	1-oz. bag	162
(*Doo Dads*—Nabisco)	1 piece	2
(*Escort*—Nabisco)	1 piece	20
(*Flings*, cheese—Nabisco)	1 piece	11
(*Flings*, Swiss 'n ham—Nabisco)	1 piece	10
(*Goldfish*—Pepperidge Farm)	5 pieces	14
Graham:		
(Nabisco)	1 piece	30
Chocolate or cocoa-covered:		
(Keebler)Deluxe	1 piece	42
(Nabisco)	1 piece	55
(Nabisco-*Fancy*)	1 piece	68
(Nabisco-*Pantry*)	1 piece	62
(*Sweet-Tooth*—Sunshine)	1 piece	45
Sugar-honey coated		
(Nabisco-*Honey Maid*)	1 piece	30
(*Hi-Ho*—Sunshine)	1 piece	18
(*Hot Potatas*—Old London)	5/8-oz. bag	82
Milk lunch (Nabisco—*Royal Lunch*)	1 piece	55
Matzo (See **MATZO**)		
Melba toast (See **MELBA**)		
Munchos	1 oz.	159
Onion flavored:		
Crisps (Snow)	1 oz.	157
French (Nabisco)	1 piece	12
(*Funyuns*—Frito-Lay)	1 oz.	137
(*Meal Mates*—Nabisco)	1 piece	19
Rings (Old London)	1/2-oz. bag	68
Rings (Wise)	1/2-oz. bag	65
Rings (Wonder)	1 oz.	133
Thins (Pepperidge Farm)	1 piece	12
Toast (Keebler)	1 piece	18
Onyums (General Mills)	10 pieces	26
OTC (Original Trenton Crackers)	1 cracker	23
Oyster:		
(Keebler)	1 piece	2
Dandy or *Oysterettes* (Nabisco)	1 piece	3
Mini (Sunshine)	1 piece	3
Peanut butter 'n cheez crackers (Kraft)	4 crackers and 3/4-oz. peanut butter	191
Peanut butter sandwich:		
Adora (Nab)	1 1/2-oz. pkg.	201
Cheese crackers (Wise)	1 piece	30
Malted Milk (Nab) 1-oz. pkg.	1 piece	34
Toasted crackers (Wise)	1 piece	30
(*Pizza Spins*—General Mills)	4 pieces	9
(*Pizza Wheels*—Wise)	3/4-oz. bag	90
Potato crisps (General Mills)	4 pieces	20
(*Ritz*, plain—Nabisco)	1 piece	16
Roman Meal Wafers	1 piece	15
Rye thins (Pepperidge Farm)	1 piece	10

Food and Description	Measure or Quantity	Calories
Rye toast (Keebler)	1 piece	17
Rye-wafers (Nabisco-*Meal Mates*)	1 piece	19
Ry-Krisp:		
Seasoned	1 triple cracker	26
Traditional	1 triple cracker	24
Saltine:		
(*Krispy*-Sunshine)	1 piece	11
(*Premium*-Nabisco; *Zesta*-Keebler)	1 piece	12
Sea toast (Keebler)	1 piece	62
Sesame:		
(Sunshine-*La Lanne*)	1 piece	15
Buttery flavored (Nabisco)	1 piece	16
Wafer (Keebler)	1 piece	16
Wafer (Nabisco-*Meal Mates*)	1 piece	21
(*Sip 'N Chips*-Nabisco)	1 piece	9
(*Sociables*-Nabisco)	1 piece	10
Soda:		
(Nabisco-*Premium*)	1 piece	12
(Sunshine)	1 piece	20
Soya (Sunshine-*La Lanne*)	1 piece	16
(*Star Lites*-Wise)	1 cup	63
Swedish rye wafer (Keebler)	1 piece	5
Taco corn chips (Old London)	1¼-oz. bag	167
Taco tortilla chips (Wonder)	1 oz.	144
Toasty (Austin's)	1 piece	37
Tortilla Chips:		
Regular, *Doritos*	1 oz.	137
Taco flavor, *Doritos*	1 oz.	150
(Old London)	1½-oz. bag	207
(Wonder)	1 oz.	148
Town House	1 piece	18
(*Triangle Thins*-Nabisco)	1 piece	8
(*Triscuit*-Nabisco)	1 piece	21
(*Twigs*, sesame & cheese-Nabisco)	1 piece	14
(*Uneeda Biscuit*-Nabisco)	1 piece	22
(*Wafer-ets*-Hol-Grain):		
Rice	1 piece	12
Wheat	1 piece	7
(*Waldorf*-Keebler)	1 piece	14
(*Waverly wafer*-Nabisco)	1 piece	18
Wheat chips (General Mills)	4 pieces	24
Wheat thins (Nabisco)	1 piece	9
Wheat toast (Keebler)	1 piece	16
(*Whistles*-General Mills)	4 pieces	17
White thins (Pepperidge Farm)	1 piece	12
Whole-wheat, natural (Froumine)	1 piece	46
CRANAPPLE (Ocean Spray)		
Regular	½ cup	94
Low calorie	½ cup	19
Frozen	½ cup	91
CRANBERRY, fresh (Ocean Spray)	1 oz.	15

Food and Description	Measure or Quantity	Calories
CRANBERRY JUICE COCKTAIL (Ocean Spray):		
Regular	½ cup	83
Low calorie	½ cup	24
Frozen	½ cup	75
CRANBERRY-ORANGE JUICE DRINK (Ocean Spray)	½ cup	67
CRANBERRY-ORANGE RELISH (Ocean Spray)	4 oz.	209
CRANBERRY PIE (Tastykake)	4-oz. pie	376
CRANBERRY SAUCE (Ocean Spray):		
Jellied	2 oz.	92
Whole berry	2 oz.	96
CRANBREAKER MIX (Bar-Tender's)	1 serving	70
CRANPRUNE (Ocean Spray)	½ cup	82
CRAZY BONE (Drake's)	1-oz. cake	115
CREAM:		
Half & Half:		
(Dean)	1 T.	22
10.5% fat (Sealtest)	1 T.	18
12% fat (Sealtest)	1 T.	20
12.8% fat (Meadow Gold)	1 T.	30
Light, table or coffee:		
16% fat (Sealtest)	1 T.	26
18% fat (Sealtest)	1 T.	28
25% fat (Sealtest)	1 T.	37
Light whipping, 30% fat (Sealtest)	1 T.	44
Heavy whipping (Dean)	1 T.	51
Sour:		
(Axelrod)	¼ of 8-oz. container	108
(Borden; Breakstone; Dean)	1 T.	28
Half & Half (Sealtest)	1 T.	20
Imitation:		
(Sealtest)	1 T.	30
(*Sour Treat*–Delite)	1 T.	25
(*Zest*–Borden)	1 T.	24
Sour dairy dressing (Sealtest)	1 T.	22
Sour dressing (Breakstone)	1 T.	27
CREAMIES (Tastykake):		
Banana cake	1⅞-oz. pkg.	238
Chocolate	1⅞-oz. pkg.	290
Koffee Kake	1⅞-oz. pkg.	303
Vanilla	1⅞-oz. pkg.	292

Food and Description	Measure or Quantity	Calories
CREAM PUFF WITH CUSTARD FILLING	3½" x 2"	303
CREAM OF RICE, cereal	4 oz.	82
CREAMSICLE (Popsicle Industries)	2½ fl. oz.	78
CREAM SOFT DRINK:		
Sweetened:		
(Canada Dry)	8 fl. oz.	129
(Clicquot Club; Cott; Mission)	8 fl. oz.	117
(Dr. Brown's; Key Food; Nedick's; Shasta; Waldbaum)	8 fl. oz.	112
(Fanta)	8 fl. oz.	125
(Hoffman; Yukon Club)	8 fl. oz.	113
(Salute)	8 fl. oz.	108
Low calorie:		
(Clicquot Club; Cott; Mision)	8 fl. oz.	4
(Dr. Brown's; Hoffman; Key Food; Waldbaum; Yukon Club)	8 fl. oz.	1
(No-Cal)	8 fl. oz.	3
(Shasta)	8 fl. oz.	<1
CREAM SUBSTITUTE:		
Coffee-mate; Cremora; Pream	1 tsp.	11
Coffee-mate	1 packet	17
Coffee Rich; Perx	1 tsp.	8
Coffee Twin	½ fl. oz.	15
Half & Half (Meadow Gold)	1 tsp.	9
N-Rich	1 tsp.	10
Poly Perx	½ oz.	20
(Sanna)	1 plastic cup	24
CREAM OF WHEAT, cereal:		
*Instant	¾ cup	99
Mix 'n Eat, dry:		
Regular	3½ T.	99
Baked apple & cinnamon	3¾ T.	129
Maple & brown sugar	3¾ T.	128
*Quick	¾ cup	99
*Regular	¾ cup	102
CREME DE ALMOND (DeKuyper)	1½ fl. oz.	156
CREME DE BANANA (DeKuyper)	1½ fl. oz.	135
CREME DE CACAO:		
(Bols)	1½ fl. oz.	152
(DeKuyper) white	1½ fl. oz.	132
(Garnier)	1½ fl. oz.	146
(Hiram Walker)	1½ fl. oz.	156
(Leroux) brown	1½ fl. oz.	152
(Leroux) white	1½ fl. oz.	147
(Old Mr. Boston)	1½ fl. oz.	126
(Old Mr. Boston)	1½ fl. oz.	142

Food and Description	Measure or Quantity	Calories
CREME DE CAFE (Leroux)	1½ fl. oz.	156
CREME DE CASSIS		
(DeKuyper)	1½ fl. oz.	142
(Garnier)	1½ fl. oz.	124
(Leroux)	1½ fl. oz.	132
CREME DE MENTHE		
(Bols)	1½ fl. oz.	183
(DeKuyper)	1½ fl. oz.	125
(Garnier)	1½ fl. oz.	165
(Hiram Walker)	1½ fl. oz.	141
(Leroux) green	1½ fl. oz.	165
(Leroux) white	1½ fl. oz.	152
(Old Mr. Boston)	1½ fl. oz.	99
(Old Mr. Boston)	1½ fl. oz.	141
CRISPY RICE, cereal	1 cup	109
CROAKER, Atlantic, baked	3 oz.	113
CUCUMBER:		
Eaten with skin	½ lb.	32
Pared, 10-oz. cucumber	7½" x 2" pared cucumber	29
Pared	3 slices	4
CUPCAKE:		
Chocolate (Tastykake)	1 cupcake	192
Chocolate, chocolate-creme filled (Tastykake)	1 cupcake	128
Chocolate, cream-filled (Drake's)	1 cupcake	187
Coconut (Tastykake)	1 cupcake	92
Creme-filled, chocolate buttercream (Tastykake)	1 cupcake	161
Devil's food cake (Hostess)	1 cupcake	162
Golden, cream-filled (Drake's)	1 cupcake	172
Lemon creme-filled (Tastykake)	1 cupcake	124
Orange (Hostess)	1 cupcake	166
Orange creme-filled (Tastykake)	1 cupcake	133
Raisin Snack (Drake's):		
Junior	1.1-oz. cake	112
Small	2¼-oz. cake	233
Vanilla creme-filled (Tastykake)	1 cupcake	123
Vanilla (*Triplets*–Tastykake)	1 cupcake	101
*****CUPCAKE MIX**, Devil's Food or yellow (Pillsbury)	1 cupcake	170
CURAÇAO		
(Bols)	1½ fl. oz.	158
(Garnier)	1½ fl. oz.	150
(Hiram Walker)	1½ fl. oz.	144

Food and Description	Measure or Quantity	Calories
CURRANT, dried, Zante (Del Monte)	¼ cup	105
CURRANT JELLY (Smucker's)	1 T.	50
CUSTARD:		
Chilled (Sealtest)	4 oz.	149
Frozen (See **ICE CREAM**)		
CUSTARD PIE:		
(Banquet)	5-oz. serving	274
(Mrs. Smith's)	⅛ of 8″ pie	296
***CUSTARD PUDDING MIX** (Royal)	½ cup	132

D

Food and Description	Measure or Quantity	Calories
DAIQUIRI COCKTAIL:		
(Hiram Walker) 52½ proof	3 fl. oz.	177
(National Distillers–*Duet*, 12½% alcohol	3 fl. oz.	105
(Party Tyme) 12½% alcohol	3 fl. oz.	98
Banana (Party Tyme) 12½% alcohol	3 fl. oz.	99
Dry mix (Bar-Tender's)	⅝-oz. serving	70
Dry mix (Holland House)	1 serving	69
Dry mix, banana:		
(Holland House)	1 serving	66
(Party Tyme)	1 serving	52
Liquid mix, canned:		
(Holland House)	2 fl. oz.	101
(Party Tyme)	2 fl. oz.	81
Liquid mix, canned, banana:		
(Holland House)	2 fl. oz.	148
(Party Tyme)	2 fl. oz.	59
DANDELION GREENS, boiled	½ cup	30
DATE:		
Whole (Cal-Date)	1 date	62
Imported Iraq (Bordo)	1 average date	18
DELAWARE WINE (Great Western)	1 fl. oz.	25
DESSERT CUP (Del Monte)	5-oz. container	173
DEVIL DOGS (Drake's):		
Regular	1 cake	178
Senior	1 cake	244

Food and Description	Measure or Quantity	Calories
DEVIL'S FOOD CAKE:		
(Pepperidge Farm)	1/8 of cake	326
Layers only (Mrs. Smith's)	1/8 of 16-oz. cake	248
*DEVIL'S FOOD CAKE MIX:		
(Duncan Hines)	1/12 of cake	205
(Swans Down)	1/12 of cake	184
Butter (Betty Crocker)	1/12 of cake	269
Red Devil (Pillsbury)	1/12 of cake	210
DING DONG (Hostess)	1 cake	185
DINNER, frozen (See individual listings such as **BEEF, CHINESE** or **ENCHILADA,** etc.)		
DIP:		
Bacon & horseradish:		
(Borden)	1 oz.	58
(Breakstone)	2 T.	62
Bacon & smoke (Sealtest–*Dip 'n Dressing*)	1 oz.	47
Barbecue (Borden)	1 oz.	58
Blue cheese:		
(Breakstone)	2 T.	64
(Dean–*Tang*)	1 oz.	61
(Kraft–*Teez*)	1 oz.	51
Chipped beef (Sealtest-*Dip 'n Dressing*)	1 oz.	46
Clam & lobster (Borden)	1 oz.	58
Cucumber & onion (Breakstone)	2 T.	55
Dill pickle (Kraft-*Ready Dip*)	1 oz.	67
Garden spice (Borden)	1 oz.	66
Garlic (Dean)	1 oz.	58
Jalapeño bean (Fritos)	1 oz.	34
Onion:		
(Borden)	1 oz.	58
(Breakstone)	2 T.	58
(Dean)	1 oz.	58
(Kraft) *Ready Dip*	1 oz.	68
Pizza (Borden)	1 oz.	58
Shrimp (Kaukauna Klub)	1 oz.	53
(*Skinny Dip*–Dean)	1 oz.	27
Tasty tartar or Western Bar B-Q (Borden)	1 oz.	48
DIP MIX:		
Bacon-onion or bleu cheese (Fritos)	1 pkg.	47
Chili con queso (Fritos)	1 pkg.	72
Green onion (Fritos)	1 pkg.	49
Guacamole (Lawry's)	1 pkg.	60
Toasted onion (Fritos; Lawry's)	1 pkg.	47
Taco (Fritos)	1 pkg.	43

Food and Description	Measure or Quantity	Calories
DISTILLED LIQUOR any proof:		
80 proof	1 fl. oz.	65
86 proof	1 fl. oz.	70
90 proof	1 fl. oz.	74
94 proof	1 fl. oz.	77
100 proof	1 fl. oz.	83
DOUGHNUT:		
(Hostess) 10 to pkg.	1¼-oz. piece	139
Cruller (Van de Kamp's)	1.5-oz. piece	161
Chocolate, Long John (Van de Kamp's)	2.1-oz. piece	179
Powdered, frozen (Morton)	1 piece	82
Sugar & spice, frozen (Morton)	1 piece	82
Yeast-leavened	2 oz.	235
DRAMBUIE (Hiram Walker)	1½ fl. oz.	165
DR. BROWN'S CEL-RAY TONIC:		
Regular	8 fl. oz.	88
Low calorie	8 fl. oz.	1
DREAMSICLE (Popsicle Industries)	3 fl. oz.	87
DR. PEPPER:		
Regular	8 fl. oz.	94
Sugar free	8 fl. oz.	3

E

Food and Description	Measure or Quantity	Calories
ECLAIR, with custard filling and chocolate icing	4 oz.	271
EEL, smoked, meat only	3 oz.	280
EGG BEATERS (Fleischmann's)	¼ cup	100
EGG, CHICKEN:		
Boiled	1 large egg	81
Fried in butter	1 large egg	99
Omelet, mixed with milk and cooked in fat	1 large egg	107
Poached	1 large egg	78
Scrambled, mixed with milk and cooked in fat	1 large egg	111
EGG McMUFFIN (McDonald's)	1 piece	313
EGG MIX (Durkee):		
Scrambled, plain	1 pkg.	124
Scrambled, with bacon	1 pkg.	181
Western omelet	1 pkg.	171

Food and Description	Measure or Quantity	Calories
EGG NOG:		
Dairy:		
(Borden) 6% fat	½ cup	154
(Borden) 8% fat	½ cup	175
(Dean)	½ cup	166
(Meadow Gold) 6% fat	½ cup	164
(Sealtest) 6% butterfat	½ cup	174
(Sealtest) 8% butterfat	½ cup	192
With alcohol (Old Mr. Boston) 30 proof	1 fl. oz.	83
EGGPLANT:		
Boiled	4 oz.	22
Frozen, fried slices (Mrs. Paul's)	7-oz. pkg.	564
Frozen, parmesan (Mrs. Paul's)	½ of 11-oz. pkg.	288
EGG ROLL:		
Chicken (Chun King)	½-oz. roll	28
Chicken & mushroom (Mow Sang)	1 roll	69
Lobster & meat (Chun King)	½-oz. roll	26
Meat & shrimp (Chun King)	½-oz. roll	29
Pork, barbecue (Mow Sang)	1 roll	74
Shrimp (Chun King)	½-oz. roll	24
Shrimp (Hung's)	1 roll	131
Shrimp (Mow Sang)	1 roll	64
EGG, SCRAMBLED, breakfast (Swanson):		
With coffee cake	6½-oz. breakfast	507
With link sausage & coffee cake	5½-oz. breakfast	409
***EGGSTRA** (Tillie Lewis)	1 large egg	43
ELDERBERRY JELLY (Smucker's)	1 T.	49
ENCHILADA, BEEF with CHEESE & CHILI GRAVY (Banquet)	1 enchilada	162
ENCHILADA DINNER:		
Beef:		
(Banquet)	12-oz. dinner	479
(Morton)	12-oz. dinner	524
(Patio) 3-compartment	13-oz. dinner	320
Cheese:		
(Banquet)	12-oz. dinner	282
(Patio) 3-compartment	12-oz. dinner	330
(Rosarita)	12-oz. dinner	436
ENCHILADA SAUCE MIX:		
(Durkee)	1 pkg.	89
* (Durkee)	1 cup	57
ENDIVE, CURLY OR ESCAROLE, cut up	½ cup	7

Food and Description	Measure or Quantity	Calories

F

FARINA:
(H-O) dry	¼ cup	162
*(Quaker)	1 cup	100

FAT, cooking, *Light Spry* — 1 T. — 93

FIG:
Small	1½" fig	30
Candied (Bama)	1 T.	37
Canned,		
heavy syrup:		
(Del Monte)	½ cup	104
(Stokely-Van Camp)	½ cup	100
Unsweetened, solids & liq.:		
Kadota (Diet Delight)	½ cup	76
(Tillie Lewis)	½ cup	64
Dried:		
Calimyrna (Del Monte)	½ cup	193
Mission (Del Monte)	½ cup	190

FIG JUICE, *Real Fig* — ½ cup — 61

FILBERT, shelled — 1 oz. — 180

FISH CAKE, (Mrs. Paul's) — 2-oz. cake — 105

FISH & CHIPS:
(Gorton)	½ of 1-lb. pkg.	395
(Mrs. Paul's)	½ of 14-oz. pkg.	353
(Swanson)	5-oz. pkg.	268

FISH CHOWDER, New England (Snow) — 8 oz. — 144

FISH DINNER:
(Morton)	8¾-oz. dinner	374
Filet of ocean fish (Swanson)	11½-oz. dinner	397
With French fries	9¾-oz. dinner	429
With green beans & perch (Weight Watchers)	18-oz. dinner	266
With pineapple chunks (Weight Watchers)	9½-oz. luncheon	175

FISH FILLET, breaded (Mrs. Paul's) — 2-oz. piece — 104

FISH FILLET SANDWICH (McDonald's) — 1 sandwich — 407

FISH PUFFS (Gorton) — ½ of 8-oz. pkg. — 265

FISH STICK, 3¾" x 1" x ½" — 15 sticks — 200

Food and Description	Measure or Quantity	Calories
FLAN, chilled (Breakstone)	5-oz. container	185
FLOUNDER:		
Baked	4 oz.	229
Dinner (Weight Watchers)	18-oz. dinner	269
& broccoli (Weight Watchers)	9½-oz. luncheon	170
FLOUR (Presto) self-rising	¼ cup	98
FOUR FRUIT PRESERVE (Smuckers's)	1 T.	52
FRANKFURTER:		
(Armour Star) all meat	1.6-oz. frankfurter	155
(Eckrich)	1.2-oz. frankfurter	112
(Hormel)	1.6-oz. frankfurter	140
(Hygrade-*Ball Park*)	2-oz. frankfurter	177
(Oscar Mayer)	1.6-oz. frankfurter	142
(Oscar Mayer) 1883	2.7-oz. frankfurter	217
(Oscar Mayer)	1.6-oz. frankfurter	143
(Wilson)	1.6-oz. frankfurter	136
(Wilson) skinless	1.6-oz. frankfurter	140
Canned (Hormel)	¼ of 12-oz. can	242
FRANKS-N-BLANKETS (Durkee)	1 piece	45
FRENCH TOAST (Aunt Jemima)	1.5-oz. slice	88
FRESCA	8 fl. oz.	<1
FROOT LOOPS (Kellogg's)	1 cup	115
FROSTED RICE KRINKLES (Post)	⅞ cup	111
FROSTED SHAKE (Borden)	9¼-fl.-oz. can	320
FROSTED TREAT (Weight Watchers)	4¾-oz. serving	140
FROSTI DEVILS (Drake's)	1 piece	164
FROZEN DESSERT:		
Charlotte Freeze (Borden):		
Chocolate	⅓ pt.	150
Vanilla	⅓ pt.	138
Chocolate:		
(Borden)	⅓ pt.	164
Chocolate chip, mint (Borden)	⅓ pt.	177
(SugarLo) 4.6% fat, ice milk	⅓ pt.	140
(SugarLo) 10.8% fat, ice cream	⅓ pt.	197
Coffee, lemon chiffon or maple (SugarLo):		
4% fat, ice milk	⅓ pt.	129
10% fat, ice cream	⅓ pt.	187

Food and Description	Measure or Quantity	Calories
Orange-pineapple or strawberry (SugarLo):		
3.6% fat, ice milk	⅓ pt.	124
9% fat, ice cream	⅓ pt.	174
Vanilla:		
(Borden)	⅓ pt.	160
Vanilla, chocolate spin (Borden)	⅓ pt.	172
FRUIT CAKE, home recipe:		
Dark	2" x 2" x ½" slice	114
Light	2" x 2" x ½" slice	117
FRUIT COCKTAIL:		
Heavy syrup (Dole)	½ cup	94
Heavy syrup (Hunt's)	½ cup	89
Dietetic pack:		
(Diet Delight)	½ cup	67
(Tillie Lewis)	½ of 8-oz. can	44
FRUIT CUP (Del Monte):		
Fruit cocktail or peaches	5¼-oz. container	106
Mixed fruits	5-oz. container	100
Pineapple	4¼-oz. container	68
FRUIT DOODLE (Drake's):		
Apple	1⅝-oz. pie	178
Cherry	1⅝-oz. pie	173
FRUITIFORT	1 oz.	111
FRUIT, MIXED (Birds Eye)	½ cup	111
FRUIT, MIXED, JELLY (Smucker's)	1 T.	49
FRUIT PUNCH (Alegre)	8 fl. oz.	130
FRUIT SALAD:		
Bottled (Kraft)	4 oz.	57
Heavy syrup (Del Monte):		
Fruits for salad	½ cup	78
Tropical	½ cup	110
Canned, dietetic pack:		
(Diet Delight)	½ cup	67
(S and W-*Nutradiet*)	4 oz.	40
FRUIT-SICLE (Popsicle Industries)	2½ fl. oz.	59
FRUITY PEBBLES (Post)	⅞ cup	111
FUDGE CAKE MIX:		
* (Pillsbury)	1/12 of cake	210
* Dark chocolate (Betty Crocker)	1/12 of cake	198
* Marble (Pillsbury)	1/12 of cake	350
* Nut (Pillsbury-*Bundt*)	1/12 of cake	300

Food and Description	Measure or Quantity	Calories
FUDGE ICE BAR:		
(Sealtest)	2½-fl.-oz. bar	91
(*Fudgsicle*–Popsicle Industries)	2½-fl.-oz. bar	102
FUNNY BONES (Drake's)	1¼-oz. cake	153
*****FUNNY FACE**, punch	8 fl. oz.	80

G

Food and Description	Measure or Quantity	Calories
GARLIC, powder (Gilroy)	1 tsp.	10
GATORADE	8 fl. oz.	70
GAZPACHO SOUP (Crosse & Blackwell)	½ of 13-oz. can	61
GEFILTE FISH (Manischewitz):		
1-lb. jar	2.2-oz. piece	60
Whitefish & pike, 1-lb. jar	1.5-oz. piece	35
(Rokeach) liquid broth:		
27-oz. can	3⅓-oz. portion	47
1-lb. or 1½-lb. can	4-oz. portion	55
1½-lb. can	6-oz. portion	83
(Rokeach) *Old Vienna*:		
27-oz. can	3⅓-oz. portion	63
1-lb. or 1½-lb. can	4-oz. portion	74
1½-lb. can	6-oz. portion	111
*****GELATIN DESSERT:**		
(Jells Best; Jell-O)	½ cup	80
(Royal)	½ cup	82
Dietetic (Dia-Mel)	1 envelope	19
Dietetic (D-Zerta)	½ cup	8
GELATIN DRINK (Knox):		
Grapefruit or orange	1 envelope	30
Plain	1 envelope	25
GEL CUP (Del Monte):		
Lemon-lime with pineapple	5-oz. container	115
Orange with peaches	5-oz. container	107
Strawberry with peaches	5-oz. container	111
GERMAN DINNER (Swanson)	11-oz. dinner	405
GEVREY-CHAMBERTIN (Cruse)	1 fl. oz.	24
GEWURZTRAMINER WINE (Wilm)	1 fl. oz.	22
GIMLET COCKTAIL:		
Canned (Party Tyme) 17½% alcohol	3 fl. oz.	123

Food and Description	Measure or Quantity	Calories
Dry mix (Holland House)	1 serving	69
Dry mix (Party Tyme)	½-oz. serving	50
Liquid mix, canned (Holland House; Party Tyme)	2 fl. oz.	80
GIN, SLOE:		
(Bols)	1½ fl. oz.	128
(DeKuyper)	1½ fl. oz.	105
(Old Mr. Boston)	1½ fl. oz.	75
GIN & TONIC, canned (Party Tyme) 10% alcohol	2 fl. oz.	55
GINGER ALE, soft drink:		
Sweetened:		
(Canada Dry; Cott; Fanta; Mission; Yukon Club)	8 fl. oz.	82
(Dr. Brown's; Key Food; Nedick's; Waldbaum)	8 fl. oz.	80
(Schweppes; Shasta)	8 fl. oz.	86
Low calorie:		
(Canada Dry; Clicquot Club; Cott; Mission; No-Cal)	8 fl. oz.	3
(Dr. Brown's; Hoffman; Key Food; Waldbaum; Yukon Club)	8 fl. oz.	1
(Shasta)	8 fl. oz.	<1
GINGERBREAD MIX (Pillsbury)	3″ sq.	190
GOOD HUMOR:		
Chocolate eclair	1 piece	224
Strawberry shortcake	1 piece	179
Toasted almond	1 piece	229
Vanilla	1 piece	197
Whammy, assorted	1 piece	136
GOOSE, roasted, meat only	3 oz.	301
GOULASH DINNER (Chef Boy-Ar-Dee)	7⅓-oz. pkg.	262
GRANOLA:		
(Pillsbury)	¼ cup	120
Vita-Crunch	¼ cup	148
Coconut & cashew (Pillsbury)	¼ cup	140
Honey almond, *Sun Country*	¼ cup	124
Raisin & almond (Pillsbury)	¼ cup	120
GRAPE:		
American type (slipskin)	3½″ x 3″ bunch	43
European type (adherent skin)	5 grapes	13
GRAPEADE, chilled (Sealtest)	8 fl. oz.	128

Food and Description	Measure or Quantity	Calories
GRAPE BERRY JUICE DRINK		
(Ocean Spray)	8 fl. oz.	184
GRAPE DRINK, sweetened:		
(Del Monte)	8 fl. oz.	120
(Hi-C)	8 fl. oz.	130
(Wagner)	8 fl. oz.	129
*GRAPE DRINK MIX (Wyler's)	8 fl. oz.	85
GRAPE JAM (Smucker's)	1 T.	52
GRAPE JELLY:		
Sweetened (Smucker's)	1 T.	50
Low calorie:		
(Louis Sherry; Smucker's)	1 T.	6
(Slenderella)	1 T.	26
GRAPE JUICE:		
(Heinz)	5½-fl.-oz. can	130
* (Minute Maid; Snow Crop)	½ cup	66
GRAPE-NUTS (Post)	¼ cup	104
GRAPE-NUTS FLAKES (Post)	⅔ cup	101
GRAPE PIE (Tastykake)	4-oz. pie	369
GRAPE SOFT DRINK:		
Sweetened:		
(Canada Dry)	8 fl. oz.	126
(Dr. Brown's; Key Food; Waldbaum)	8 fl. oz.	116
(Fanta; Grapette)	8 fl. oz.	122
(Hoffman; Nedick's; Nehi; Yukon Club)	8 fl. oz.	124
(Patio)	8 fl. oz.	128
(Salute; Yoo Hoo-high protein)	8 fl. oz.	134
(Shasta)	8 fl. oz.	117
Low calorie:		
(Dr. Brown's, Hoffman; Key Food; No-Cal; Waldbaum)	8 fl. oz.	3
(Shasta; Yukon Club)	8 fl. oz.	<1
GRAPEFRUIT:		
Pink & red:		
Seeded type	½ med. grapefruit	46
Seedless type	½ med. grapefruit	49
White:		
Seeded type	½ med. grapefruit	44
Seedless type	½ med. grapefruit	46
Bottled, sweetened (Kraft)	4 oz.	53
Bottled, unsweetened (Kraft)	4 oz.	40
Canned, syrup pack:		
(Del Monte)	½ cup	69

Food and Description	Measure or Quantity	Calories
(Stokely-Van Camp)	½ cup	88
Canned, unsweetened		
(Diet Delight)	½ cup	41
GRAPEFRUIT DRINK:		
Sweetened (Wagner)	8 fl. oz.	114
Low calorie (Wagner)	8 fl. oz.	16
GRAPEFRUIT JUICE:		
Fresh, pink, red or white,		
California or Arizona	½ cup	52
Fresh, pink, red or white, Florida	½ cup	46
Bottled, sweetened (Kraft)	½ cup	60
Bottled, unsweetened (Kraft)	½ cup	48
Canned:		
Sweetened (Heinz)	5½-fl.-oz. can	73
Unsweetened (Heinz)	5½-fl.-oz. can	56
*Frozen, unsweetened (Minute Maid; Snow Crop)	½ cup	50
GRAPEFRUIT SOFT DRINK:		
Sweetened:		
(Clicquot Club; Cott; Mission)	8 fl. oz.	110
(Fanta)	8 fl. oz.	112
(Hoffman; Shasta)	8 fl. oz.	108
(Salute)	8 fl. oz.	106
Low calorie:		
(Canada Dry; Shasta)	8 fl. oz.	<1
(Clicquot Club; Cott; Mission)	8 fl. oz.	4
(Hoffman; No-Cal) pink	8 fl. oz.	3
GRASSHOPPER COCKTAIL MIX (Holland House)	1 serving	69
GRAVES WINE (B & G; Cruse)	1 fl. oz.	23
GRAVY:		
Beef (Franco-American)	¼ cup	44
Brown, *Ready Gravy*	¼ cup	44
Mushroom:		
(B in B)	¼ cup	44
Brown, *Dawn Fresh*	½ of 5¾-oz. can	30
(Franco-American)	¼ cup	27
GRAVY MIX:		
Au jus (Durkee)	1 pkg.	67
*Brown (French's)	¼ cup	18
Chicken (Durkee)	1 pkg.	96
*Chicken (Pillsbury)	¼ cup	30
Mushroom (Durkee)	1 pkg.	60
Onion (Durkee)	1 pkg.	85
GRAVY with MEAT or TURKEY:		
Beef chunks (Bunker Hill)	½ of 15-oz. can	394

Food and Description	Measure or Quantity	Calories
Frozen:		
Giblet & sliced turkey (Banquet)	5-oz. bag	129
Sliced beef (Morton House)	½ of 12½-oz. can	189
Sliced pork (Morton House)	½ of 12½-oz. can	193
Sliced turkey (Morton House)	½ of 12½-oz. can	140
GUAVA	1 guava	48
GUAVA JELLY (Smucker's)	1 T.	50

H

Food and Description	Measure or Quantity	Calories
HADDOCK:		
Fried, breaded	4" x 3" x ½" fillet	165
Smoked	3 oz.	88
HADDOCK MEALS:		
(Banquet)	8¾-oz. dinner	419
(Weight Watchers)	18-oz. dinner	256
& spinach (Weight Watchers)	9½-oz. luncheon	175
HALIBUT, broiled	6½" x 2½" x ⅝" steak	214
HAM:		
Boiled:		
(Hormel)	1 oz.	35
Chopped, sliced (Hormel)	1 oz.	70
Minced (Oscar Mayer)	.8-oz. slice	56
Smoked (Oscar Mayer)	.7-oz. slice	29
Canned (Swift)	5" x 2¼" x ¼" slice	111
Canned (Swift–*Hostess*)	1 oz.	41
Deviled:		
(Armour Star)	1 oz.	79
(Hormel)	1 oz.	73
(Libby's)	1 oz.	83
(Underwood)	¼ of 4½-oz. can	110
HAM & CHEESE LOAF (Oscar Mayer)	1-oz. slice	69
HAM CROQUETTE	3 oz.	213
HAM DINNER:		
(Banquet)	10-oz. dinner	369
(Morton)	10½-oz. dinner	447
*Mix, au gratin (Jeno's)	¼ of 35-oz. pkg.	407
HAM SPREAD (Oscar Mayer)	1 oz.	60
HAMBURGER (McDonald's):		
Regular	1 hamburger	251
Big Mac (See **BIG MAC**)		

Food and Description	Measure or Quantity	Calories
Cheese, regular	1 hamburger	310
¼ pound	1 hamburger	416
Cheese, ¼ pound	1 hamburger	523
HAWAIIAN PUNCH	8 fl. oz.	120
HEADCHEESE (Oscar Mayer)	1-oz. slice	52
HEARTLAND, cereal	1 oz.	122
HERRING, canned:		
Bismarck, drained (Vita)	5-oz. jar	273
Cocktail, drained (Vita)	8-oz. jar	342
In cream sauce (Vita)	8-oz. jar	397
HERRING, smoked, kippered	3 oz.	179
HICKORY NUT, shelled	1 oz.	191
HOB NOB, any flavor (Drake's)	1 piece	68
HO-HO (Hostess)	1-oz. cake	133
HOMINY GRITS:		
Dry (Pocono)	1 oz.	101
Cooked (Aunt Jemima/Quaker)	⅔ cup	100
HONEY, strained	1 T.	61
HONEYDEW	2" x 7" wedge	31
HORSERADISH:		
Regular (Kraft)	1 oz.	3
Cream style (Kraft)	1 oz.	9
HUSH PUPPY, refrigerated (Borden)	1 piece	58

I

ICE CREAM & FROZEN CUSTARD: (See also listing by flavor or brand name or **FROZEN DESSERT**):		
Candy, 11% fat (Dean)	¼ pt.	180
Chocolate, 11.7% fat (Dean)	¼ pt.	176
Frozen custard, 10% fat (Dean)	¼ pt.	128
Fruit, 10.4% fat (Dean)	¼ pt.	168
Nut, 14% fat (Dean)	¼ pt.	188
Strawberry, 10.5% fat (Dean)	¼ pt.	168
Vanilla, 10.1% fat (Dean)	¼ pt.	148
Vanilla, 12% fat (Dean)	¼ pt.	170

Food and Description	Measure or Quantity	Calories
ICE CREAM BAR, chocolate-coated:		
(Popsicle Industries)	3-fl.-oz. bar	180
(Sealtest)	2½-fl.-oz. bar	149
ICE CREAM CONE, cone only:		
(Comet)	1 piece	19
Rolled sugar (Comet)	1 piece	49
ICE CREAM CUP, cup only		
(Comet)	1 piece	20
ICE CREAM SANDWICH		
(Sealtest)	3 fl. oz.	173
ICE MILK:		
Hardened	¼ pt.	100
Soft-serve	¼ pt.	83
Any flavor (Borden) 2.5% fat	¼ pt.	93
Any flavor (Borden) 3.25% fat	¼ pt.	97
(*Count Calorie*–Dean)	¼ pt.	78
5% fat (Dean)	¼ pt.	113
(*Light n' Lively*–Sealtest):		
Buttered almond	¼ pt.	117
Chocolate	¼ pt.	105
Coffee, lemon or vanilla	¼ pt.	102
Strawberry	¼ pt.	100
Vanilla fudge royale	¼ pt.	113
ICE MILK BAR, chocolate-coated:		
(Popsicle Industries)	3-fl.-oz. bar	133
(Sealtest)	2½-fl.-oz. bar	132
ICE STICK, Twin Pops (Sealtest)	3 fl. oz.	70
ITALIAN DINNER:		
(Banquet)	11-oz. dinner	446
(Swanson)	13½-oz. dinner	448

J

Food and Description	Measure or Quantity	Calories
JACK ROSE MIX (Bar-Tender's)	1 serving	70
JOHANNISBERG RIESLING (Inglenook)	1 fl. oz.	20

K

Food and Description	Measure or Quantity	Calories
KABOOM (General Mills)	1 cup	109

Food and Description	Measure or Quantity	Calories
KALE:		
Boiled, leaves only	4 oz.	44
Chopped (Birds Eye)	½ cup	29
KARO, pancake & waffle syrup	1 T.	60
KIELBASA (Eckrich)	1 link	184
KING VITAMIN (Quaker)	¾ cup	118
KIX (General Mills)	1½ cups	112
KNOCKWURST		
(Oscar Mayer) *Chubbies*	2.4-oz. link	210
****KOOL-AID*** (General Foods):*		
Regular	1 cup	98
Sugar-sweetened	1 cup	91
KOOL-POPS (General Foods)	1.5-oz. bar	32
KUMQUAT, flesh & skin	4 oz.	74

L

Food and Description	Measure or Quantity	Calories
LAMB:		
Leg:		
Roasted, lean & fat	3 oz.	237
Roasted, lean only	3 oz.	158
Loin. One 5-oz. chop (weighed with bone before cooking) will give you:		
Lean & fat	2.8 oz.	280
Lean only	2.3 oz.	122
Rib. One 5-oz. chop (weighed with bone before cooking) will give you:		
Lean & fat	2.9 oz.	334
Lean only	2 oz.	118
Shoulder:		
Roasted, lean & fat	3 oz.	287
Roasted lean only	3 oz.	174
LAMB STEW, canned (B & M)	½ cup	96
LASAGNE:		
Canned (Chef Boy-Ar-Dee)	⅛ of 40-oz. can	279
Frozen (Buitoni)	½ of 15-oz. pkg.	255
Frozen (Celeste)	¼ of 2-lb. pkg.	413
Mix (Golden Grain)	⅕ of 7-oz. pkg.	151
*Mix, dinner (Jeno's)	¼ of 30-oz. pkg.	400
LAZY BONE (Drake's)	.9-oz. cake	94
LEMONADE:		
Chilled (Sealtest)	8 fl. oz.	110

Food and Description	Measure or Quantity	Calories
Frozen:		
* (Minute Maid; Snow Crop)	8 fl. oz.	98
*Low calorie (Weight Watchers)	8 fl. oz.	11
*Mix (Wyler's)	8 fl. oz.	85
LEMON EXTRACT (Virginia Dare)	1 tsp.	22
LEMON JUICE:		
(Sunkist)	1 lemon	11
ReaLemon	1 T.	3
LEMON-LIME DRINK (Wagner)	8 fl. oz.	114
LEMON-LIME SOFT DRINK:		
Sweetened (Salute)	8 fl. oz.	96
Low calorie, *Diet Rite*	8 fl. oz.	3
LEMON PIE:		
(Hostess)	4½-oz. pie	447
(Tastykake)	4-oz. pie	336
Frozen:		
(Mrs. Smith's)	⅙ of 8″ pie	340
Cream (Banquet)	2½-oz. serving	179
Cream (Morton)	⅙ of 16-oz. pie	194
Cream (Mrs. Smith's)	⅙ of 8″ pie	227
Krunch (Mrs. Smith's)	⅙ of 8″ pie	383
Meringue (Mrs. Smith's)	⅙ of 8″ pie	261
Tart (Pepperidge Farm)	3-oz. pie tart	317
LEMON PIE FILLING (Wilderness)	⅙ of 22-oz. can	184
LEMON PUDDING, canned:		
(Hunt's)	5-oz. can	175
(Thank You)	½ cup	183
***LEMON PUDDING or PIE MIX** (Royal)	⅛ of 9″ pie (includes crust)	224
LEMON SOFT DRINK, sweetened:		
(Canada Dry-*Hi-Spot*)	8 fl. oz.	96
(Royal Crown)	8 fl. oz.	118
LEMON TURNOVER (Pepperidge Farm)	1 turnover	341
LENTIL SOUP:		
* (Manischewitz)	½ cup	83
With ham (Crosse & Blackwell)	½ of 13-oz. can	123
Mix (Lipton-*Cup-a-Soup*)	1 pkg.	123
LETTUCE:		
Bibb or Boston	4″ head	23
Cos or Romaine, shredded or broken into pieces	½ cup	4

Food and Description	Measure or Quantity	Calories
Grand Rapids, Salad Bowl or Simpson	2 large leaves	9
Iceberg, New York or Great Lakes, leaves	½ cup	4
LIEBFRAUMILCH WINE:		
(Anheuser)	1 fl. oz.	21
(Deinhard) Hans Christof	1 fl. oz.	20
(Deinhard) lilac seal	1 fl. oz.	20
(Julius Kayser) Glockenspiel	1 fl. oz.	19
LIFE, cereal (Quaker)	⅔ cup	107
LIKE, soft drink	8 fl. oz.	1
LIME	1 med. lime	15
*LIMEADE (Minute Maid; Snow Crop)	½ cup	50
LIME JUICE, *ReaLime*	1 T.	2
LIME PIE, Key lime, cream (Banquet)	2½-oz. serving	204
LIME PIE FILLING:		
Canned (Comstock)	⅙ of 8" pie	144
*Mix, Key lime (Royal)	⅛ of 9" pie (including crust)	222
LIVER:		
Beef, fried	6½" x 2⅜" x ⅜" slice	195
Calf, fried	6½" x 2⅜" x ⅜" slice	222
Chicken, simmered	2" x 2" x ⅝" liver	41
LIVERWURST, sliced (Oscar Mayer)	.9-oz. slice	95
LIVERWURST SPREAD (Underwood)	1 tsp.	15
LOBSTER:		
Cooked, meat only	1 cup	138
Canned, meat only	4 oz.	108
Frozen, South African lobster tail:		
3 in 8-oz. pkg.	1 piece	87
4 in 8-oz. pkg.	1 piece	65
5 in 8-oz. pkg.	1 piece	51
LOBSTER NEWBURG, frozen (Stouffer's)	½ of 11½-oz. pkg.	336
LOBSTER PASTE, canned	1 oz.	51
LOBSTER SALAD	4 oz.	125

Food and Description	Measure or Quantity	Calories
LOBSTER SOUP:		
Bisque (Lipton-*Cup-a-Soup*)	1 pkg.	104
Cream of (Crosse & Blackwell)	½ of 13-oz. can	92
LOG CABIN, syrup, regular	1 T.	46
LOQUAT, fresh, flesh only	2 oz.	27
LOVE BIRD COCKTAIL MIX (Holland House)	1 serving	69
LUNCHEON MEAT (See also individual listings, e.g., **BOLOGNA**):		
All meat (Oscar Mayer)	1-oz. slice	98
Bar-B-Que loaf (Oscar Mayer)	1-oz slice	48
Beef, chopped (Eckrich-*Slender Sliced*)	1 oz.	38
Chicken, chipped (Eckrich-*Slender Sliced*)	1 oz.	77
Chicken breast loaf (Eckrich)	1 oz.	32
Cocktail loaf (Oscar Mayer)	1-oz. slice	62
Gourmet loaf (Eckrich)	1-oz. slice	38
Ham, chipped, smoked (Eckrich-*Slender Sliced*)	1 oz.	47
Ham & cheese (See **HAM & CHEESE**)		
Honey loaf (Eckrich)	1 slice	42
Honey loaf (Oscar Mayer)	1-oz. slice	40
Jellied:		
Beef loaf (Oscar Mayer)	1-oz. slice	41
Corned beef loaf (Oscar Mayer)	1-oz. slice	39
Luncheon loaf (Sugardale)	1-oz. slice	77
Luncheon roll, sausage, all meat (Oscar Mayer)	.8-oz. slice	27
(*Luxury Loaf*–Oscar Mayer)	1-oz. slice	40
Meat loaf	1 oz.	57
Minced roll sausage, all meat (Oscar Mayer)	.8-oz. slice	54
Old-fashioned loaf:		
(Oscar Mayer)	1-oz. slice	62
(Sugardale)	1-oz. slice	76
Olive loaf (Oscar Mayer)	1-oz. slice	62
Peppered loaf (Eckrich)	1 oz.	38
Peppered loaf (Oscar Mayer)	1-oz. slice	46
Pickle & pimento:		
(Hormel)	1-oz.	81
(Oscar Mayer)	1-oz. slice	62
(Sugardale)	1-oz. slice	78
Picnic loaf (Oscar Mayer)	1 oz. slice	64
Plain loaf (Oscar Mayer)	1-oz. slice	75
Pork loin, chipped, smoked (Eckrich-*Slender Sliced*)	1-oz.	40
Pressed luncheon loaf (Eckrich)	1-oz.	40

Food and Description	Measure or Quantity	Calories
Pure beef (Oscar Mayer)	1-oz. slice	75
Spiced (Hormel)	1 oz.	70
Turkey, chipped, smoked (Eckrich-*Slender Sliced*)	1 oz.	38

M

Food and Description	Measure or Quantity	Calories
MACADAMIA NUT (Royal Hawaiian)	¼ cup	394
MACARONI, cooked:		
8-10 minutes, firm	1 cup	192
14-20 minutes, tender	1 cup	155
MACARONI & BEEF:		
Canned:		
Tiny meatballs & sauce (Buitoni)	4 oz.	111
In tomato sauce (Franco-American)	½ cup	112
Frozen, with tomatoes (Stouffer's)	½ of 11½-oz. pkg.	205
MACARONI & CHEESE:		
Canned:		
(Franco-American)	1 cup	219
(Heinz)	8¼-oz. can	231
Frozen:		
(Banquet)	8 oz. bag	279
(Kraft)	½ of 12½-oz. pkg.	306
(Morton)	½ of 20-oz. pkg.	368
(Stouffer's)	½ of 12-oz. pkg.	238
Mix, dinner (Golden Grain)	¼ of 7¼-oz. pkg.	202
MACARONI DINNER, frozen:		
& beef:		
(Banquet)	12-oz. dinner	394
(Morton)	11-oz. dinner	287
& cheese:		
(Banquet)	12-oz. dinner	326
(Morton)	12¾-oz. dinner	384
MACARONI SALAD, canned (Nalley's)	4 oz.	203
MACKEREL, Atlantic, broiled with fat	8½" x 2½" x ½" fillet	248
MADEIRA WINE (Leacock)	1 fl. oz.	40
MAI TAI COCKTAIL:		
Canned:		
(Lemon Hart) 48 proof	3 fl. oz.	180
(National Distillers-*Duet*) 12% alcohol	8-fl.-oz. can	288

Food and Description	Measure or Quantity	Calories
(Party Tyme) 12½% alcohol	3 fl. oz.	98
Dry mix: (Bar-Tender's; Holland House)	1 serving	69
(Party Tyme)	½-oz. serving	50
Liquid mix, canned (Holland House)	2 fl. oz.	67
MALTED MILK MIX:		
Chocolate (Horlicks)	3 heaping tsps.	124
Natural (Horlicks)	3 heaping tsps.	127
MALT LIQUOR, *Champale*	8 fl. oz.	122
***MALT-O-MEAL**, chocolate	¾ cup	102
MANDARIN ORANGE:		
Light syrup (Del Monte)	½ cup	77
(Diet Delight; S & W-*Nutradiet*)	½ cup	54
MANGO, fresh, diced	1 med. mango	88
MANGO DRINK:		
(Yoo-Hoo) high protein	8 fl. oz.	133
& pineapple (Alegre)	8 fl. oz.	186
MANHATTAN COCKTAIL:		
Canned:		
(Hiram Walker) 55 proof	3 fl. oz.	147
(National Distillers-*Duet*) 20% alcohol	8-fl. oz. can	576
(Party Tyme) 20% alcohol	3 fl. oz.	111
Brandy (National Distillers-*Duet*) 20% alcohol	8-fl. oz. can	560
Dry mix (Bar-Tender's)	1 serving	24
Liquid mix, canned (Holland House)	2 fl. oz.	59
MANICOTTI DINNER, fresh (Celeste)	2 manicotti with sauce	428
MAPLE SYRUP:		
(Cary's)	1 T.	63
Dietetic (Tillie Lewis)	1 T.	3
MARGARINE:		
Regular	1 oz.	204
Regular	1 T.	101
Regular	1 pat (1″ x ⅓″ x 1″, 5 grams)	36
MARGARINE, IMITATION:		
(Fleischmann's; Mazola)	1 T.	50
(Parkay)	1 T.	55
MARGARINE, WHIPPED (Blue Bonnet; Miracle; Parkay)	1 T.	67

Food and Description	Measure or Quantity	Calories
MARGARITA COCKTAIL:		
Canned:		
(National Distillers-*Duet*)		
12½% alcohol	8-fl.-oz. can	248
(Party Tyme) 12½% alcohol	3 fl. oz.	99
Dry Mix:		
(Bar-Tender's; Holland House)	1 serving	70
(Party Tyme)	½-oz. serving	50
Liquid Mix:		
(Holland House)	2 fl. oz.	77
(Party Tyme)	2 fl. oz.	63
MARGAUX (B & G)	1 fl. oz.	21
MARINADE MIX, chicken or meat		
(Adolf's)	1 tsp.	8
MARMALADE:		
Sweetened:		
(Bama; Smucker's)	1 T.	54
(Crosse & Blackwell)	1 T.	60
Low calorie:		
(S and W-*Nutradiet*)	1 T.	11
(Slenderella)	1 T.	22
MARTINI COCKTAIL:		
Gin:		
(Hiram Walker) 67.5 proof	3 fl. oz.	168
(National Distillers-*Duet*),		
21% alcohol	8-fl.-oz. can	560
(Party Tyme) 24% alcohol	3 fl. oz.	123
Liquid mix (Holland House)	2 fl. oz.	20
Liquid mix (Party Tyme)	2 fl. oz.	12
Vodka:		
(Hiram Walker) 60 proof	3 fl. oz.	147
(National Distillers-*Duet*)		
20% alcohol	8-fl.-oz. can	536
(Party Tyme) 21% alcohol	3 fl. oz.	72
MATZO:		
Regular (Manischewitz)	1 matzo	114
Diet-10's (Goodman's)	1 small square	12
Egg (Manischewitz)	1 matzo	133
Tea (Goodman's)	1 matzo	70
Unsalted (Goodman's)	1 matzo	109
MAYONNAISE:		
(Best Foods–*Real*; Hellmann's–*Real*)	1 T.	102
(Dia-Mel)	1 T.	99
Saffola	1 T.	92
MAY WINE (Deinhard)	3 fl. oz.	60
MEATBALL, cocktail (Cresca)	1 meatball	10

Food and Description	Measure or Quantity	Calories
MEATBALL STEW (Morton House)	1 cup	295
MEAT LOAF DINNER:		
(Banquet)	11-oz. dinner	412
(Morton) 3-course	15½-oz. dinner	656
(Swanson)	10¾-oz. dinner	419
MEAT LOAF ENTREE:		
(Banquet)	5-oz. bag	281
In brown gravy (Morton House)	⅛ of 12½-oz. can	178
In tomato sauce (Morton House)	⅛ of 12½-oz. can	188
MEAT TENDERIZER (Adolf's)	1 tsp.	2
MELBA TOAST, salted:		
Garlic, onion or plain (Keebler)	1 piece	9
Garlic or onion rounds (Old London)	1 piece	10
Pumpernickel, wheat or white (Old London)	1 piece	17
Sesame (Keebler)	1 piece	11
Sesame round (Old London)	1 piece	11
MELON BALL, in syrup, frozen	½ cup	72
MEXICAN DINNER, frozen:		
Combination:		
(Banquet)	12-oz. dinner	571
(Patio)	11-oz. dinner	380
Mexican style:		
(Banquet)	16-oz. dinner	608
(Morton)	14-oz. dinner	409
(Patio) 3-compartment	12-oz. dinner	270
(Swanson) 3-course	18-oz. dinner	613
MILK, CONDENSED, *Dime Brand; Eagle Brand; Magnolia Brand*	1 T.	60
*MILK, DRY, nonfat, instant (Carnation; Sanalac)	1 cup	81
MILK, EVAPORATED (Carnation):		
Regular	1 T.	22
Skim	1 T.	12
MILK, FRESH:		
Whole, 3.5% fat (Dean)	1 cup	151
Skim:		
0.5% fat (Dean)	1 cup	91
1.0% fat (Dean)	1 cup	103
2.0% fat (Dean)	1 cup	133
(*Light n' Lively*–Sealtest)	1 cup	114
(*Lite-Line*–Borden)	1 cup	119
(*Pro-Line*–Borden)	1 cup	140
(*Skim-Line*–Borden)	1 cup	99

Food and Description	Measure or Quantity	Calories
(*Vita-Lure*–Sealtest)	1 cup	137
(*Viva*–Meadow Gold)	1 cup	137
Buttermilk:		
(Dean)	1 cup	95
1.0% fat (Borden)	1 cup	107
(*Light n' Lively*–Sealtest)	1 cup	95
Chocolate milk:		
With whole milk (Dean)	1 cup	212
With skim milk, 1% fat (Dean)	1 cup	166
With skim milk, 0.5% fat (Sealtest)	1 cup	146
MILK SHAKE (McDonald's):		
Chocolate	1 serving	318
Strawberry	1 serving	313
Vanilla	1 serving	324
MINCEMEAT (Wilderness)	⅛ of 22-oz. can	215
MINCE PIE:		
(Banquet)	5-oz. serving	401
(Morton)	⅙ of 24-oz. pie	297
(Mrs. Smith's)	⅙ of 8" pie	339
(Tastykake)	4-oz. pie	373
MINESTRONE SOUP:		
* (Campbell)	1 cup	82
(Crosse & Blackwell)	½ of 13-oz. can	107
MINT LEAVES	½ oz.	4
***MOCHA NUT PUDDING MIX** (Royal)	½ cup	199
MOLASSES (Grandma's)	1 T.	60
MOUNTAIN DEW, soft drink	8 fl. oz.	122
MR. PIBB, soft drink	8 fl. oz.	93
MRS. BUTTERWORTH'S SYRUP	1 T.	53
MUFFIN:		
Blueberry, frozen (Morton)	1.6-oz. muffin	116
Blueberry, frozen (Mrs. Smith's)	.9-oz. muffin	116
Bran (Thomas') with raisins	1.9-oz. muffin	170
Corn:		
(Morton) frozen	1.7-oz. muffin	132
(Mrs. Smith's) frozen	1-oz. muffin	157
(Thomas')	2-oz. muffin	194
English:		
(Arnold)	2.2-oz. muffin	145
(Newly Weds)	2.5-oz. muffin	167
(Thomas')	2.1-oz. muffin	140
Scone (*Raisin Round*–Wonder)	2-oz. piece	147

Food and Description	Measure or Quantity	Calories
Sour dough (Wonder)	2-oz. muffin	133
Wheat Berry (Wonder)	2-oz. muffin	136
MUFFIN MIX, corn (Albers)	1 oz.	118
MUSCATEL WINE:		
(Gallo)	1 fl. oz.	29
(Gold Seal)	1 fl. oz.	53
(Taylor)	1 fl. oz.	49
MUSHROOM:		
Raw slices (Shady Oaks)	½ cup	10
Canned in butter (B & B)	6-oz. can	50
Canned (Shady Oaks)	4-oz. can	19
Dried	1 oz.	72
Frozen, in butter sauce (Green Giant)	⅓ pkg.	30
MUSHROOM SOUP:		
Bisque (Crosse & Blackwell)	½ of 13-oz. can	103
Cream of:		
*(Campbell)	½ cup	66
*(Heinz)	½ cup	62
(Heinz-*Great American*)	½ cup	66
MUSHROOM SOUP MIX:		
*Beef flavor (Lipton)	½ cup	20
Cream of (Wyler's)	1 pkg.	78
MUSTARD:		
(French's; Gulden's; *Grey Poupon*)	1 tsp.	6
Horseradish (Best Foods)	1 tsp.	4
Salad (French's)	1 tsp.	4
Yellow (Heinz)	1 tsp.	5
MUSTARD GREENS, boiled, drained	½ cup	26

N

NATURAL CEREAL:		
100% (Quaker)	¼ cup	140
100% with fruit (Quaker)	¼ cup	136
NEAPOLITAN CREAM PIE, frozen:		
(Banquet)	2½-oz. serving	188
(Morton)	⅙ of 16-oz. pie	198
(Mrs. Smith's)	⅛ of 8" pie	244
NECTARINE, flesh only	4 oz.	73
NIAGARA WINE, white (Pleasant Valley)	1 fl. oz.	28

Food and Description	Measure or Quantity	Calories
NOODLE, 1½″ strips, cooked	1 cup	200
NOODLE CHOW MEIN (Chun King)	1 cup	211
NOODLE MIX, Parmesano, Noodle-Roni	⅕ of 6-oz. pkg.	130
NUT, MIXED:		
Dry roasted:		
(Flavor House)	1 oz.	172
(Planters)	1 oz.	176
(Skippy)	1 oz.	168
Oil roasted:		
With peanuts (Planters)	1 oz.	176
Without peanuts (Planters)	1 oz.	178

O

Food and Description	Measure or Quantity	Calories
OAT FLAKES (Post)	⅔ cup	107
OATMEAL:		
Dry, instant (H-O):		
Sweet & mellow	1 packet	149
With dates & caramel	1 packet	147
With raisins & spice	1 packet	167
*Cooked, old fashioned (Quaker)	⅔ cup	107
OCEAN PERCH:		
Fried	3 oz.	193
Dinner:		
(Banquet)	8¾-oz. dinner	434
(Weight Watchers)	18-oz. dinner	307
& broccoli (Weight Watchers)	9½-oz. luncheon	185
OIL, SALAD OR COOKING		
Corn (Fleischmann's; Mazola)	1 T.	126
Olive or soybean	1 T.	124
Peanut (Planters)	1 T.	126
(Saffola; Wesson)	1 T.	124
OKRA, whole (Birds Eye)	½ cup	27
OLD FASHIONED:		
Cocktail (Hiram Walker) 62 proof	3 fl. oz.	165
Dry mix (Bar-Tender's)	1 serving	20
Liquid mix (Holland House)	2 fl. oz.	72
OLIVE:		
Green	4 med. or 3 extra large or 2 giant	19
Ripe, Mission	3 small or 2 large	18

Food and Description	Measure or Quantity	Calories
ONION:		
Raw, slices	½ cup	21
Boiled, pearl onions	½ cup	27
Dehydrated, flakes (Gilroy)	1 tsp.	6
French-fried rings:		
Battered (Mrs. Paul's)	⅓ of 9-oz. pkg.	189
Breaded (Mrs. Paul's)	⅓ of 9-oz. pkg.	254
Pickled, cocktail (Crosse & Blackwell)	1 T.	1
Small with cream sauce (Birds Eye)	⅓ pkg.	132
ONION, GREEN	1 small onion	3
ONION SOUP:		
*(Campbell)	½ cup	20
(Crosse & Blackwell)	½ of 13-oz. can	46
(Hormel)	½ of 15-oz. can	72
ONION SOUP MIX:		
*(Lipton)	½ cup	17
(Lipton-*Cup-a-Soup*)	1 pkg.	30
ORANGE:		
Whole	1 med. orange	77
Sections	½ cup	59
ORANGEADE, chilled (Sealtest)	½ cup	64
ORANGE-APRICOT JUICE DRINK (Del Monte)	8 fl. oz.	157
ORANGE CREAM BAR (Sealtest)	2½-fl.-oz. bar	103
ORANGE DRINK		
Bottled (Wagner)	8 fl. oz.	114
*Crystals (Wagner)	8 fl. oz.	120
Island orange (Alegre)	8 fl. oz.	136
ORANGE-GRAPEFRUIT JUICE:		
Bottled, chilled (Kraft)	½ cup	60
*Frozen (Minute Maid; Snow Crop)	½ cup	51
ORANGE ICE (Sealtest)	¼ pt.	130
ORANGE JUICE:		
Chilled (Kraft)	½ cup	60
Chilled (Minute Maid)	½ cup	55
Sweetened (Heinz)	5½-fl.-oz. can	91
Unsweetened (Heinz)	5½-fl.-oz. can	71
*Frozen (Nature's Best)	½ cup	58
ORANGE PEEL, candied (Liberty)	1 oz.	93
ORANGE-PINEAPPLE DRINK (Wagner)	8 fl. oz.	114

Food and Description	Measure or Quantity	Calories
ORANGE-PINEAPPLE PIE (Tastykake)	4-oz. pie	374
ORANGE PUDDING (Royal-*Creamerino*)	5-oz. container	225
ORANGE SOFT DRINK:		
Sweetened:		
(Canada Dry; *Orangette*)	8 fl. oz.	125
(Clicquot Club; Cott; Mission)	8 fl. oz.	137
(Dr. Brown's; Fanta; Nedicks; Waldbaum)	8 fl. oz.	121
(Hoffman)	8 fl. oz.	124
(Key Food)	8 fl. oz.	114
(Kirsch; White Rock)	8 fl. oz.	117
(Nehi; Salute)	8 fl. oz.	133
(Patio)	8 fl. oz.	128
(Shasta; Yukon Club)	8 fl. oz.	126
(Yoo-Hoo) high protein	8 fl. oz.	133
Low calorie:		
(Canada Dry; Shasta)	8 fl. oz.	<1
(Cliquot Club; Cott; Mission; No-Cal)	8 fl. oz.	3
(*Diet Rite;* Dr. Brown's; Hoffman; Key Food; Nedick's; Waldbaum; Yukon Club)	8 fl. oz.	1
OYSTER:		
Raw:		
Eastern	19-31 small or 13-19 med.	158
Pacific & Western	6-9 small or 4-6 med.	218
Canned, solids & liq. (Bumble Bee)	3 oz.	64
Fried	3 oz.	203
OYSTER STEW, home recipe	½ cup	103

P

Food and Description	Measure or Quantity	Calories
*PANCAKE MIX, complete (Pillsbury):		
Blueberry, *Hungry Jack*	4" pancake	120
Buttermilk, *Hungry Jack*	4" pancake	73
PANCAKE & WAFFLE SYRUP (Smucker's)	1 T.	62
PAPAYA, fresh:		
Cubed	½ cup	36
Juice	4 oz.	78
PARSLEY, CHOPPED	1 T.	2

Food and Description	Measure or Quantity	Calories
PASSION FRUIT, Giant, whole	1 lb.	53
PASTRAMI (Vienna)	1-oz. slice	57
PASTRY SHELL:		
Pot pie (Keebler)	4″ shell	236
Tart (Keebler)	3″ shell	158
PÂTÉ:		
De foie gras	1 T.	69
Liver (Sell's)	1 T.	45
PEA:		
Boiled	½ cup	58
Canned, solids & liq., *April Showers*	½ of 8½-oz. can	65
Canned, Early June, with onion (Green Giant)	¼ of 17-oz. can	67
In butter sauce, sweet (Green Giant)	⅓ pkg.	86
In butter sauce, early, *Le Sueur*	⅓ pkg.	78
With cream sauce (Birds Eye)	⅓ pkg.	125
With cream sauce (Green Giant)	⅓ pkg.	66
PEA & CARROT:		
Canned (Del Monte)	½ cup	38
Frozen, in cream sauce (Green Giant)	⅓ pkg.	60
PEA & ONION, in butter sauce (Green Giant)	⅓ pkg.	75
PEA POD, boiled	4 oz.	49
PEA & POTATO, with cream sauce (Birds Eye)	⅓ pkg.	131
PEA SOUP, green:		
* (Campbell)	½ cup	66
* (Lipton)	½ cup	69
(Lipton-*Cup-a-Soup*)	1 pkg.	127
PEA SOUP, split:		
*With ham (Campbell)	½ cup	80
*With ham (Heinz)	½ cup	76
PEACH:		
Fresh, whole	2½″ piece	38
Fresh, slices	½ cup	32
Canned heavy syrup:		
(Hunt's)	½ cup	96
Spiced (Del Monte)	½ cup	96
Canned, dietetic pack:		
(Diet Delight)	½ cup	61
(Tillie Lewis) cling	½ of 8-oz. can	43
Dried (Del Monte)	½ cup	199
Frozen (Birds Eye)	½ cup	87

Food and Description	Measure or Quantity	Calories
PEACH BRANDY (DeKuyper)	1½ fl. oz.	128
PEACH BUTTER (Smucker's)	1 T.	45
PEACH CREEK		
(Annie Green Springs)	1 fl. oz.	21
PEACH LIQUEUR (DeKuyper)	1½ fl. oz.	123
PEACH PIE:		
(Banquet)	5-oz. serving	320
(Hostess)	4½-oz. pie	415
(Mrs. Smith's)	⅙ of 8″ pie	301
(Mrs. Smith's) natural juice	⅙ of 8″ pie	329
Filling (Wilderness)	⅙ of 21-oz. can	113
PEACH PRESERVE (Smucker's)	1 T.	50
PEACH TURNOVER		
(Pepperidge Farm)	1 turnover	323
PEANUT:		
Dry (Franklin)	1 oz.	163
Dry (Frito-Lay; Skippy)	1 oz.	168
Dry (Planters)	1 oz. (jar)	170
Oil (Planters)	1 oz. (can)	179
Nab	¾-oz. pkg.	134
Spanish, dry (Planters)	1 oz. (jar)	175
Spanish, oil, *Freshnut*	1 oz.	170
Spanish, oil (Planters)	1 oz. (can)	182
PEANUT BUTTER:		
(Bama) crunchy	1 T.	100
(Bama) smooth	1 T.	103
(Planters)	1 T.	100
(Skippy) chunk or creamy	1 T.	96
& raspberry (Smucker's-*Goober*)	1 T.	61
PEANUT SPREAD, diet (Peter Pan)	1 T.	100
PEAR:		
Whole	3″ x 2½″ pear	101
Canned, heavy syrup	2 med. halves & 2 T. syrup	89
Canned, dietetic (Tillie Lewis)	½ of 8-oz. can	44
Dried (Del Monte)	½ cup	178
PECAN	6-7 halves	48
PECAN PIE, frozen:		
(Morton)	⅙ of 16-oz. pie	275
(Mrs. Smith's)	⅙ of 8″ pie	430
PEP, cereal	¾ cup	103

Food and Description	Measure or Quantity	Calories
PEPPER:		
Black	1 tsp.	4
Lemon (Durkee)	1 tsp.	1
Seasoned (Lawry's)	1 tsp.	8
PEPPER, HOT CHILI, canned (Del Monte)	¼ cup	11
PEPPER, STUFFED:		
Home recipe	2¾" x 2½" pepper with 1⅛ cups stuffing	314
Frozen, with veal (Weight Watchers)	12-oz. dinner	224
PEPPER, SWEET:		
Green, whole	½ med.	6
Red, whole	1 med.	19
PERCH, BREADED (Gorton)	⅓ of 11-oz. pkg.	113
PERNOD (Julius Wile)	1½ fl. oz.	118
PERSIMMON	4.4-oz. persimmon	81
PICKLE:		
Cucumber, fresh or bread & butter (Aunt Jane's)	1 slice or stock	5
Dill, *L & S*	1 large pickle	15
Dill, candied (Smucker's)	4" pickle	46
Kosher dill (Smucker's)	3½" pickle	8
Sour (Heinz)	2" pickle	1
Sweet:		
Gherkin (Bond's)	1 pickle	19
Mixed (Heinz)	1 piece	8
*****PIECRUST MIX** (Pillsbury)	⅛ of 2-crust pie	290
PIGS FEET, pickled (Hormel)	½ cup	110
PILLSBURY INSTANT BREAKFAST, chocolate	1 pouch	130
PIMM'S CUP, scotch (Julius Wile)	1½ fl. oz.	102
PIÑA COLADA:		
(Party Tyme) 12½% alcohol	3 fl. oz.	94
Dry mix (Holland House)	1 serving	66
Dry mix (Party Tyme)	½-oz. pkg.	50
Liquid mix (Holland House)	2 fl. oz.	120
PINEAPPLE:		
Chunks (Dole)	½ cup	52
Slices in pineapple juice (Dole)	2 med. slices & 2½ T. juice	66
Canned, chunks:		
Juice pack (Dole)	½ of 8-oz. can	64

Food and Description	Measure or Quantity	Calories
Heavy syrup (Dole)	½ of 8-oz. can	84
PINEAPPLE & GRAPEFRUIT JUICE DRINK (Wagner)	8 fl. oz.	114
PINEAPPLE JUICE:		
(Heinz)	5½-fl. oz can	101
(Stokely-Van Camp)	½ cup	63
PINEAPPLE PIE:		
(Hostess)	4½-oz. pie	415
Frozen, with cheese (Mrs. Smith's)	⅙ of 8" pie	263
PINEAPPLE PRESERVE (Smucker's)	1 T.	52
PINEAPPLE SOFT DRINK (Hoffman; Kirsch; Nedick's)	8 fl. oz.	118
PINE NUT, pignolias, shelled	1 oz.	156
PINK SQUIRREL COCKTAIL MIX (Holland House)	1 serving	69
PINOT CHARDONAY (Inglenook)	1 fl. oz.	19
PINOT NOIR (Inglenook)	1 fl. oz.	19
PISTACHIO NUT:		
In shell	½ cup	197
Shelled	¼ cup	184
PIZZA PIE:		
With cheese:		
(Celeste-*Bambino*)	¼ or 10-oz, pie	158
(Buitoni)	4 oz.	270
(Celeste)	⅙ of 20-oz. pie	214
(Chef Boy-Ar-Dee)	⅙ of 12½-oz. pie	131
Little (Chef Boy-Ar Dee)	2½-oz. pie	162
(Jeno's)	⅙ of 13-oz. pie	147
(Jeno's-*Serv-A-Slice*)	1.7-oz. slice	116
(Jeno's-*Snack Tray*)	½-oz. pizza	30
(Kraft)	⅙ of 14-oz. pie	138
(Kraft-*Pee Wee*)	2½-oz. pizza	169
(Lambrecht)	⅙ of 13-oz. pie	152
With hamburger (Jeno's)	⅙ of 13½-oz. pie	154
With pepperoni:		
(Buitoni)	2 oz.	144
(Chef Boy-Ar-Dee)	⅙ of 14-oz. pie	150
(Jeno's)	⅙ of 13¼-oz. pie	168
(Jeno's-*Serv-A-Slice*)	1.8-oz. slice	145
(Jeno's-*Snack Tray*)	½-oz. pizza	37
With sausage:		
(Buitoni)	2 oz.	140
(Celeste)	⅛ of 23-oz. pie	200

Food and Description	Measure or Quantity	Calories
(Celeste-*Bambino*)	¼ of 9-oz. pie	160
(Chef Boy-Ar-Dee)	⅙ of 13¼-oz. pie	141
(Jeno's)	⅙ of 13½-oz. pie	150
Little (Chef Boy-Ar-Dee)	2½-oz. pie	168
(Jeno's)	⅙ of 13½-oz. pie	145
(Jeno's-*Serv-A-Slice*)	2-oz. slice	143
(Jeno's-*Snack Tray*)	½-oz. pizza	35
(Kraft)	⅙ of 14½-oz. pie	166
(Kraft-*Pee Wee*)	2½-oz. pizza	191
(Lambrecht)	⅙ of 14-oz. pie	168
PIZZA PIE MIX:		
Regular	⅙ of 14-oz. pkg.	160
With cheese:		
(Chef Boy-Ar-Dee)	⅙ of 15½-oz. pie	156
(Jeno's)	⅙ of 14¾-oz. pkg.	183
(Kraft)	2 oz.	133
With pepperoni (Jeno's)	⅙ of 14¾-oz. pkg.	210
With sausage:		
(Jeno's)	⅙ of 16½ oz. pkg.	207
(Kraft)	2 oz.	137
PIZZA ROLL:		
Cheeseburger (Jeno's) 12 to pkg.	½-oz. roll	44
Pepperoni (Jeno's) 12 to pkg.	½-oz. roll	42
Sausage (Jeno's) 12 to pkg.	½-oz. roll	42
Shrimp (Jeno's) 12 to pkg.	½-oz. roll	35
Snack Tray (Jeno's):		
Hamburger	½-oz. roll	41
Pepperoni	½-oz. roll	38
Sausage	½-oz. roll	39
PLUM:		
Japanese & hybrid, fresh	2" plum	27
Prune-type, fresh, halves	½ cup	60
Canned (Stokely-Van Camp)	½ cup	100
Canned, dietetic (Tillie Lewis)	½ of 8-oz. can	61
PLUM JELLY OR PRESERVE (Smucker's)	4-oz. pie	364
PLUM PUDDING (Richardson & Robbins)	½ cup	300
POLISH-STYLE SAUSAGE, Kolbase (Hormel)	1 oz.	80
POMEGRANATE, pulp only	4 oz.	71
POMMARD WINE (B & G)	1 fl. oz.	22
POPCORN:		
Buttered (Jiffy Pop)	½ of 5-oz. pkg.	247

Food and Description	Measure or Quantity	Calories
Caramel-coated:		
Without peanuts (Old London)	1¾-oz. bag	195
With peanuts (Old London)	½ cup	71
Cracker Jack	1¾-oz. bag	90
Cracker Jack	1⅝-oz. box	165
Cracker Jack	3-oz. box	360
Cheese (Wise)	⅝-oz. bag	90
POPOVER	2¾″ popover	90
POPSICLE (Popsicle Industries):		
All flavors, except chocolate	3 fl. oz.	70
Chocolate	3 fl. oz.	106
PORK:		
Fresh		
Chop:		
Broiled, lean & fat	3-oz. chop (weighed without bone)	332
Broiled, lean only	3-oz. chop (weighed without bone)	230
Loin:		
Roasted, lean & fat	3 oz.	308
Roasted, lean only	3 oz.	216
Spareribs, braised	3 oz.	374
Cured ham:		
Roasted, lean & fat	3 oz.	246
Roasted, lean only	3 oz.	159
(Wilson) Festival, smoked	3 oz.	143
Picnic, canned (Hormel)	3 oz.	154
PORK DINNER (Swanson)	10-oz. dinner	460
PORK RINDS, *Baken-ets*	1 oz.	139
PORK SAUSAGE, cooked:		
Bulk style (Oscar Mayer)	1 oz.	99
(*Little Friers*–Oscar Mayer)	1 oz.	106
PORK, SWEET & SOUR (Chun King)	½ pkg. (7½ oz.)	220
PORT WINE:		
(Gallo)	1 fl. oz.	31
(Great Western) Solera	1 fl. oz.	45
(Louis M. Martini)	1 fl. oz.	55
(Robertson's) tawny	1 fl. oz.	48
POST TOASTIES (Post)	1 cup	108
***POSTUM**, instant	1 cup	16
POTATO:		
Baked, peeled	2½″ dia potato	92
Boiled, peeled	4.3-oz. potato	79

Food and Description	Measure or Quantity	Calories
French-fried (McDonald's)	1 serving	218
Hash-browned, home recipe	½ cup	223
Mashed, milk & butter added	½ cup	92
Dehydrated, mashed (Borden)	¼ cup	60
Frozen:		
Bake-A-Tata (Holloway House):		
With cheese	1 potato	226
With sour cream	1 potato	200
(Holloway House) stuffed, baked with cheese or sour cream & chives	1 potato	296
*Mix, au gratin (Pillsbury)	½ cup	170
*Mix, hash brown (Pillsbury)	½ cup	140
*Mix, mashed (Pillsbury)	½ cup	170
POTATO CHIP:		
(Lay's; *Ruffles*)	1 oz.	158
(Pringle's)	5 chips	46
(Wise)	1-oz. bag	156
Barbecue (Lay's)	1 oz.	155
Julienne (Wise)	⅝-oz. bag	98
(*Ridgies*, sour cream–Wise)	⅞-oz. bag	131
Sour cream & onion (Wise)	¾-oz. bag	113
POTATO SALAD, home recipe	½ cup	181
***POTATO SOUP** (Lipton)	½ cup	50
POTATO STICK (Durkee-*O & C*)	½ of 1½-oz. can	116
POUILLY-FUISSE WINE:		
(B & G)	1 fl. oz.	21
(Chanson) St. Vincent	1 fl. oz.	28
(Cruse)	1 fl. oz.	24
POUILLY-FUME WINE (B & G)	1 fl. oz.	20
POUND CAKE:		
(Drake's) all butter, Jr.	1.2-oz. slice	110
(Drake's) plain	1.6-oz. slice	153
(Sara Lee)	1½-oz. slice	165
*Mix (Pillsbury-*Bundt*)	½ of cake	300
PRETZEL:		
(Nabisco-*Mister Salty*, Dutch)	½-oz. piece	51
(Nabisco-*Mister Salty Veri-Thin*)	1 stick	1
(Old London) nuggets	2-oz. bag	211
Rold Gold, twists	1 oz.	100
PRODUCT 19 (Kellogg's)	1 cup	107
PRUNE:		
Dried	1 med. prune	15
Canned (Sunsweet)	½ cup	150
PRUNE JUICE, *RealPrune*	½ cup	74

Food and Description	Measure or Quantity	Calories
PRUNE WHIP, home recipe	½ cup	106
PUFFA PUFFA RICE, cereal	1 cup	120
PUFFED RICE or WHEAT (State Fair)	½ oz.	52
PULIGNY MONTRACHET WINE (B & G)	1 fl. oz.	20
PUMPKIN (Libby's)	½ cup	41
PUMPKIN PIE:		
(Morton)	⅙ of 24-oz. pie	201
(Mrs. Smith's)	⅙ of 8″ pie	242
PUMPKIN SEED	1 oz.	157

Q

QUANGAROOS, cereal (Quaker)	1 cup	112
QUININE SOFT DRINK OR TONIC WATER:		
Sweetened:		
(Canada Dry)	8 fl. oz.	90
(Dr. Brown's; Hoffman; Schweppes)	8 fl. oz.	88
(Kirsch)	8 fl. oz.	94
(Shasta)	8 fl. oz.	76
Low calorie (No-Cal)	8 fl. oz.	3

R

RADISH	2 small radishes	4
RAISIN (Sun-Maid)	1 T.	31
RAISIN PIE:		
(Mrs. Smith's)	⅙ of 8″ pie	322
Filling (Wilderness)	⅙ of 22-oz. can	129
RALSTON, cereal	¼ cup	106
RASPBERRY, fresh:		
Black	½ cup	49
Red	½ cup	41
RASPBERRY BRANDY (DeKuyper)	1½ fl. oz.	128
RASPBERRY DRINK MIX (Wyler's)	1 rounded T.	86

Food and Description	Measure or Quantity	Calories
RASPBERRY PRESERVE		
(Smucker's) red	1 T.	51
RASPBERRY SOFT DRINK:		
Sweetened:		
(Clicquot Club; Cott; Mission)	8 fl. oz.	130
(Dr. Brown's)	8 fl. oz.	114
(Hoffman; Shasta; Yukon Club)	8 fl. oz.	118
Low calorie:		
(Clicquot Club; Mission; No-Cal)	8 fl. oz.	4
(Dr. Brown's; Hoffman; Key Food; Waldbaum)	8 fl. oz.	3
(Shasta)	8 fl. oz.	<1
RAVIOLI:		
Canned:		
Meat (Prince)	3.7-oz. can	136
Cheese (Prince)	3.7-oz. can	123
Frozen:		
Beef (Celeste)	7 ravioli	259
Beef dinner (Celeste)	½ of 15-oz. pkg.	262
Cheese (Celeste)	7 ravioli	264
Cheese dinner (Celeste)	½ of 15-oz. pkg.	255
RELISH:		
Barbecue (Heinz)	1 T.	35
Corn (Crosse & Blackwell)	1 T.	15
Hamburger (Del Monte)	1 T.	33
Hot dog (Heinz)	1 T.	17
RHINESKELLER WINE		
(Italian Swiss Colony)	1 fl. oz.	22
RHINE WINE:		
(Great Western)	1 fl. oz.	24
(Inglenook) Vintage	1 fl. oz.	21
(Taylor)	1 fl. oz.	23
RHUBARB, cooked, sweetened	½ cup	169
RICE:		
Brown:		
Parboiled (Uncle Ben's) no added butter	⅔ cup	133
Frozen (Green Giant)	⅓ pkg.	128
White:		
*Instant (Minute Rice) no added butter	⅔ cup	124
*Regular, extra long-grain (Carolina)	⅔ cup	149
White & wild, frozen (Green Giant)	⅓ pkg.	104
***RICE CHEX**, cereal*	1⅛ cups	111

Food and Description	Measure or Quantity	Calories
RICE, FRIED:		
Pork, canned (Chun King)	⅔ cup	163
Shrimp, frozen (Temple)	⅔ cup	198
RICE KRISPIES (Kellogg's)	1 cup	108
RICE MIX:		
Beef, *Rice-A-Roni*	⅛ of 8-oz. pkg.	129
Chicken, *Rice-A-Roni*	⅕ of 8-oz. pkg.	153
Oriental, dinner (Jeno's)	¼ of 40-oz. pkg.	400
Spanish, *Rice-A-Roni*	⅙ of 7½ oz. pkg.	125
RICE PUDDING:		
Home recipe	½ cup	193
Canned (Hunt's)	5-oz. can	240
Spanish (Uncle Ben's) with added butter	½ cup	129
RIESLING WINE, Grey (Inglenook)	1 fl. oz.	20
RING DINGS (Drake's)	2-oz. cake	292
ROE, baked or broiled, cod & shad	3 oz.	107
ROLAIDS	1 piece	4
ROLL & BUN:		
Barbecue (Arnold)	1 bun	132
Brown & serve (Wonder)	1 roll	85
Butter crescent (Pepperidge Farm)	1 roll	127
Butter, old fashioned (Pepperidge Farm)	1 roll	36
Butterfly (Pepperidge Farm)	1 roll	58
Cinnamon nut (Pepperidge Farm)	1 bun	92
Club (Pepperidge Farm)	1 roll	114
Deli Twist (Arnold)	1 roll	115
Diet size (Arnold)	1 roll	40
Dinner (Pepperidge Farm)	1 roll	61
Dinner (Wonder)	1 roll	85
Dutch Egg, sandwich (Arnold)	1 bun	143
Finger:		
(Sara Lee)	1 oz.	84
Poppy (Pepperidge Farm)	1 roll	59
Sesame (Pepperidge Farm)	1 roll	60
Frankfurter:		
(Arnold)	1 roll	121
(Pepperidge Farm)	1 roll	117
(Wonder)	2-oz. roll	162
French:		
Butter (Van de Kamp's)	1 roll	105
Triple (Pepperidge Farm)	1 roll	253
Twin (Pepperidge Farm)	1 roll	389

Food and Description	Measure or Quantity	Calories
Golden Twist (Pepperidge Farm)	1 roll	123
Hamburger:		
(Pepperidge Farm)	1 roll	112
(Wonder)	2-oz. roll	162
Hard (Levy's)	1 roll	130
Hearth (Pepperidge Farm)	1 roll	59
Honey, frozen (Morton)	1 serving	170
Hot Cross (Van de Kamp's)	1 bun	63
Kaiser, brown & serve (Arnold)	1 roll	132
Old Fashioned (Pepperidge Farm)	1 roll	57
Parker (Arnold) handipan	1 roll	63
Parkerhouse (Pepperidge Farm)	1 roll	57
(*Party Pan*–Pepperidge Farm) plain or poppy	1 roll	34
Pecan coffee (Pepperidge Farm)	1 bun	195
Sandwich, soft (Arnold)	1 roll	135
Sesame crisp (Pepperidge Farm):		
Mid-west	1 roll	69
East	1 roll	73
Sesame seed (Sara Lee)	1 oz.	84
Soft (Arnold) handipan	1 roll	58
Sourdough, French (Van de Kamp's)	1 roll	130

ROLL DOUGH:
Butterflake (Pillsbury)	1 roll	55
Crescent (Borden)	1 roll	104

*ROLL MIX:
Cinnamon (Pillsbury)	1 roll	240
Hot (Pillsbury)	1 roll	95

*ROMAN MEAL CEREAL   ¾ cup   130

ROOT BEER, soft drink:
Sweetened:		
(Canada Dry-*Rooti*; Hire's)	8 fl. oz.	101
(Dad's)	8 fl. oz.	105
(Dr. Brown's; Fanta; Hoffman; Key Food; Nedick's; Waldbaum)	8 fl. oz.	102
(Kirsch)	8 fl. oz.	94
(Nehi)	8 fl. oz.	125
(Patio)	8 fl. oz.	110
(Salute)	8 fl. oz.	122
(Shasta) draft	8 fl. oz.	112
(Yukon Club)	8 fl. oz.	108
Low calorie:		
(Canada Dry; Clicquot Club; Cott; Dad's; Hoffman; Mission; No-Cal; Shasta; Yukon Club)	8 fl. oz.	<1

Food and Description	Measure or Quantity	Calories
ROSÉ WINE:		
(Antinori; Great Western)	1 fl. oz.	28
(Inglenook)	1 fl. oz.	21
(Mogen David)	1 fl. oz.	25
RUM & COLA (Party Tyme) 10% alcohol	3 fl. oz.	82
RUSK (Nabisco)	1 piece	49
RUTABAGA, boiled, mashed	½ cup	43
RY-KING (See **BREAD**)		
RY-KRISP (See **CRACKER**)		

S

Food and Description	Measure or Quantity	Calories
SAINT-EMILION (B & G)	1 fl. oz.	21
SAKE WINE	1 fl. oz.	39
SALAD DRESSING:		
Avocado (Marzetti)	1 T.	80
(Bama)	1 T.	59
Bennett's	1 T.	51
Blendaise (Marzetti)	1 T.	60
Bleu or blue cheese:		
(Bernstein's) Danish	1 T.	44
(Kraft) Imperial	1 T.	68
(Lawry's)	1 T.	57
Caesar (Lawry's)	1 T.	70
Coleslaw (Bernstein's)	1 T.	60
French:		
(Best Foods; Hellmann's)	1 T.	65
(Wish-Bone) Garlic	1 T.	66
Garlic, French (Hellmann's)	1 T.	68
Green Goddess:		
(Kraft)	1 T.	75
(Wish-Bone)	1 T.	68
Italian:		
(Lawry's)	1 T.	80
(Lawry's) with cheese	1 T.	60
(Wish-Bone)	1 T.	75
Miracle Whip (Kraft)	1 T.	69
Oil & vinegar (Kraft)	1 T.	65
Onion, California (Wish-Bone)	1 T.	76
Rich 'n' Tangy (Dutch Pantry)	1 T.	68
Roquefort (Marzetti)	1 T.	80
Russian (Kraft) creamy	1 T.	68
(Saffolá)	1 T.	52

Food and Description	Measure or Quantity	Calories
Sweet 'n' Sour (Dutch Pantry)	1 T.	76
Thousand Island:		
(Best Foods)	1 T.	60
(Lawry's)	1 T.	69
Tomato 'n' Spice (Dutch Pantry)	1 T.	66
Vinaigrette (Bernstein's)	1 T.	41
SALAD DRESSING, DIETETIC or LOW CALORIE:		
Bleu or blue:		
(Frenchette) chunky	1 T.	20
(Kraft; *Slimette;* Tillie Lewis)	1 T.	13
Caesar (Frenchette)	1 T.	32
Chef Style (Kraft)	1 T.	16
Chef's (Tillie Lewis)	1 T.	2
(*Diet Mayo 7*–Bennett's)	1 T.	23
French:		
(Bennett's)	1 T.	21
(Frenchette)	1 T.	9
(Tillie Lewis)	1 T.	6
Green Goddess (Slim-ette)	1 T.	12
Italian:		
(Bernstein's)	1 T.	4
(*Italian*-Frenchette)	1 T.	7
(Tillie Lewis)	1 T.	<1
(Wish-Bone)	1 T.	16
May-lo-naise (Tillie Lewis)	1 T.	16
(*Mayonette Gold*–Frenchette)	1 T.	32
Russian (Wish-Bone)	1 T.	24
Slaw (Frenchette)	1 T.	28
Thousand Island:		
(Frenchette)	1 T.	22
(Kraft)	1 T.	28
Vinaigrette (Bernstein's)	1 T.	1
Whipped (Tillie Lewis)	1 T.	16
SALAMI:		
Beef (Sugardale)	1-oz. slice	76
Cotto, all meat (Oscar Mayer)	.8-oz. slice	55
SALISBURY STEAK:		
(Swanson-*Hungry Man*)	17-oz. dinner	943
(Morton)	11-oz. dinner	343
(Morton) 3-course	15½-oz. dinner	642
SALMON:		
Baked or broiled	6¾" x 2½" x 1"	264
Pink or Humpback, canned:		
(Del Monte)	7¾-oz. can	268
(Icy Point; Pink Beauty)	7¾-oz. can	310
Sockeye or Red or Blueback:		
(Bumble Bee) including bones	1 cup	286

Food and Description	*Measure or Quantity*	*Calories*
(Icy Point; Pillar Rock)	3¾-oz. can	181
(Del Monte)	7¾-oz. can	304
SALMON SMOKED:		
Lox, drained (Vita)	4-oz. jar	136
Nova, drained (Vita)	4-oz. can	221
SALT:		
Seasoned (Morton)	1 tsp.	3
Substitute, seasoned (Adolf's)	1 tsp.	5
SANDWICH SPREAD:		
(Best Foods; Hellmann's)	1 T.	62
(Kraft)	1 oz.	105
Corned beef (Carnation)	⅕ can	96
Ham salad (Carnation)	⅕ can	90
SARDINE,		
Moroccan (Cresca):		
In olive oil	3¾-oz. can	341
In water	3¾-oz. can	165
Norwegian (Underwood):		
In mustard sauce	3¾-oz. can	196
In oil, drained	3¾-oz. can	232
In tomato sauce	3¾-oz. can	169
SAUCE:		
A-1	1 T.	12
Barbecue:		
(French's) smoky	1 T.	15
(General Foods) hickory smoke, *Open Pit*	1 T.	27
(Heinz) with onions, hickory smoke	1 T.	18
(Kraft) hickory smoke	1 oz.	34
Escoffier Sauce Diable	1 T.	16
Escoffier Sauce Robert	1 T.	20
Famous (Durkee) 6½-oz. bottle	1 T.	72
(57–Heinz)	1 T.	14
(*H.P. Steak Sauce*–Lea & Perrin)	1 T.	20
Seafood (Bernstein's)	1 T.	19
Seafood cocktail (Crosse & Blackwell)	1 T.	22
Sloppy Joe (Contadina)	1 T.	9
Soy (Chun King)	1 T.	6
Steak, mushroom, *Dawn Fresh*	⅕ of 5¾-oz. can	9
Steak Supreme (Heublein)	1 T.	20
Sweet & sour (LaChoy)	1 T.	30
Tartar (Best Foods; Hellmann's)	1 T.	71
White, medium	¼ cup	103
Worcestershire (Lea & Perrin)	1 T.	12

Food and Description	Measure or Quantity	Calories
SAUCE MIX:		
*A la King (Durkee)	¼ cup	34
*Cheese (Durkee)	¼ cup	84
*Hollandaise (Durkee)	¼ cup	52
SAUERKRAUT (Steinfeld's Western Acres)	½ of 8-oz. can	25
SAUSAGE, after browning (Swift)	1 link	88
SAUTERNES:		
(B & G)	1 fl. oz.	32
(Great Western)	1 fl. oz.	27
(Italian Swiss Colony)	1 fl. oz.	20
(Taylor)	1 fl. oz.	27
SCALLOP:		
Steamed	3 oz.	95
Breaded, fried (Mrs. Paul's)	½ of 7-oz. pkg.	206
SCHNAPPS, PEPPERMINT (DeKuyper)	1½ fl. oz.	118
SCOTCH SOUR COCKTAIL:		
(National Distillers-*Duet*) 12½% alcohol	8-fl.-oz. can	272
(Party Tyme) 12½% alcohol	3 fl. oz.	98
SCREWDRIVER:		
Canned:		
(National Distillers-*Duet*) 12½% alcohol	8-fl.-oz. can	288
(Party Tyme) 12½% alcohol	3 fl. oz.	104
Dry mix (Bar-Tender's; Holland House)	1 serving	70
SEAFOOD PLATTER, breaded, fried (Mrs. Paul's)	½ of 9-oz. pkg.	259
SENEGALESE SOUP (Crosse & Blackwell)	½ of 13-oz. can	61
SEVEN-UP:		
Regular	8 fl. oz.	97
Low Calorie	8 fl. oz.	28
SHAD, baked	3 oz.	171
SHERBET (Dean)	¼ pt.	137
SHERRY:		
Cocktail (Gold Seal)	1 fl. oz.	41
Cream:		
(Great Western) Solera	1 fl. oz.	46
(Taylor)	1 fl. oz.	50

Food and Description	Measure or Quantity	Calories
Dry:		
(ItalianSwiss Colony-Gold Medal)	1 fl. oz.	35
(Williams & Humbert)	1 fl. oz.	40
Dry Sack (Williams & Humbert)	1 fl. oz.	40
SHREDDED WHEAT:		
(Kellogg's) frost...	1 biscuit	27
(Nabisco)	1 biscuit	86
(Nabisco-*Spoon Size*)	1 piece	4
SHRIMP:		
Canned, solids & liq. (Bumble Bee)	4½-oz. can	90
Canned (Icy Point; Pillar Rock; Snow Mist)	4½-oz. can	148
Frozen, fried (Mrs. Paul's)	½ of 6-oz. pkg.	158
SHRIMP CAKE, thin (Mrs. Paul's)	2½-oz. cake	158
SHRIMP COCKTAIL:		
(Sau-Sea)	4-oz. jar	107
(Sea Snack)	4-oz. jar	110
SHRIMP DINNER (Morton)	7¾-oz. pkg.	374
SHRIMP PUFF (Durkee)	1 piece	44
SIDE CAR COCKTAIL MIX (Holland House)	2 fl. oz.	88
SIP 'N SLIM, cocktail mix (Holland House)	2 fl. oz.	19
SLENDER (Carnation):		
Dry	1 pkg.	104
Liquid	10-fl.-oz. can	225
SLIM . JIM	1 piece	83
SLOPPY JOE (Morton House)	¾ cup	251
SNO BALL (Hostess)	1 cake	162
SOAVE WINE (Antinori)	1 fl. oz.	28
SOLE:		
Dinner (Weight Watchers)	18-oz. dinner	279
& cauliflower (Weight Watchers)	9½-oz. luncheon	190
In lemon butter (Gorton)	⅓ of 9-oz. pkg.	147
SOUTHERN COMFORT		
86 proof	1 fl. oz.	84
100 proof	1 fl. oz.	96

Food and Description	Measure or Quantity	Calories
SOYBEAN CURD or TOFU	2¾" x 2½" x 1" cake	86
SOYBEAN NUT (*Soytown*)	1 oz.	145
SPAGHETTI, COOKED:		
8-10 minutes, "al dente"	1 cup	216
14-20 minutes, tender	1 cup	155
SPAGHETTI DINNER:		
(Banquet)	11½-oz. dinner	450
(Morton)	11-oz. dinner	390
(Swanson)	12-oz. dinner	323
SPAGHETTI & GROUND BEEF IN TOMATO SAUCE		
(Chef Boy-Ar-Dee)	½ of 15-oz. can	192
SPAGHETTI & MEATBALLS in TOMATO SAUCE (Morton)	½ of 20-oz. casserole	360
SPAGHETTI with MEAT SAUCE:		
(Banquet)	8-oz. bag	311
(Heinz)	8½-oz. can	207
SPAGHETTI SAUCE:		
Clam, white (Buitoni)	4 oz.	140
Italian (Contadina)	½ cup	76
Italian, frozen (Celeste)	½ cup	68
Meat:		
(Buitoni)	4 oz.	111
(Chef Boy-Ar-Dee)	4 oz.	136
Meatless:		
(Buitoni)	4 oz.	76
(Chef Boy-Ar-Dee)	4 oz.	73
Mushroom (Buitoni; Chef Boy-Ar-Dee)	4 oz.	69
SPAGHETTI with TOMATO SAUCE:		
(Van Camp)	1 cup	168
With cheese:		
Home recipe	1 cup	260
Canned (Heinz)	1 can	164
SPAM (Hormel)	1 oz.	87
SPECIAL K (Kellogg's)	1¼ cups	107
SPINACH:		
Whole leaves	½ cup	4
Boiled	½ cup	18
Frozen:		
(Birds Eye)	⅓ pkg.	23
In cream sauce (Green Giant)	⅓ pkg.	57

Food and Description	*Measure or Quantity*	*Calories*
Leaf, in butter sauce (Green Giant)	⅓ pkg.	48
SPINACH SOUFFLÉ (Stouffer's)	⅓ of 12-oz. pkg.	161
SPONGE CAKE	1/12 of 10″ cake	196
SPRITE	8 fl. oz.	93
SQUASH, SUMMER:		
Yellow, boiled, slices	½ cup	13
Zucchini, boiled, slices	½ cup	9
Canned, zucchini in tomato sauce (Del Monte)	½ cup	25
SQUASH, WINTER:		
Acorn, baked	½ cup	56
Hubbard, baked, mashed	½ cup	51
(Birds Eye)	⅓ pkg.	43
****START***	½ cup	60
STRAWBERRY:		
Fresh, capped	½ cup	26
Frozen:		
Whole (Birds Eye)	¼ pkg.	101
Halves (Birds Eye)	½ cup	162
STRAWBERRY DRINK (Hi-C)	8 fl. oz.	130
STRAWBERRY ICE CREAM:		
(Meadow Gold) 10% fat	¼ pt.	126
(Sealtest)	¼ pt.	133
STRAWBERRY PIE:		
Cream (Morton)	⅙ of 16-oz. pie	183
Cream (Mrs. Smith's)	⅙ of 8″ pie	221
Filling (Wilderness)	⅙ of 21-oz. can	123
STRAWBERRY PRESERVE:		
Sweetened (Smucker's)	1 T.	51
Low calorie; (Dia-Mel; Louis-Sherry)	1 T.	6
Low calorie (Slenderella)	1 T.	25
Low calorie (Smucker's)	1 T.	2
STRAWBERRY-RHUBARB PIE:		
(Tastykake)	4-oz. pie	399
(Mrs. Smith's) natural juice	⅙ of 9″ pie	316
STRAWBERRY SHORTCAKE (Mrs. Smith's)	⅙ of 9″ pie	379

Food and Description	Measure or Quantity	Calories
STRAWBERRY SOFT DRINKS:		
Sweetened:		
(Canada Dry; Fanta; Hoffman)	8 fl. oz.	117
(Clicquot Club; Cott; Mission)	8 fl. oz.	130
(Salute)	8 fl. oz.	128
(Shasta)	8 fl. oz.	106
(Yukon Club)	8 fl. oz.	122
Low calorie:		
(Canada Dry; Hoffman; Shasta)	8 fl. oz.	<1
(Clicquot Club; Cott; Mission)	8 fl. oz.	4
STRUDEL (Pepperidge Farm):		
Apple	1/6 of strudel	202
Blueberry	1/6 of strudel	240
Cherry	1/6 of strudel	204
Pineapple-cheese	1/6 of strudel	209
STURGEON, smoked	3 oz.	127
SUCCOTASH (Birds Eye)	1/2 cup	87
SUGAR:		
Brown	1 T.	48
Confectioners'	1 T.	30
Granulated	1 T.	46
Maple	1¾" x 1¼" x ½" piece	104
Substitute (Adolph's)	1 tsp.	14
SUGAR FROSTED FLAKES:		
(Kellogg's)	3/4 cup	108
(Ralston Purina)	3/4 cup	113
SUGAR JETS (General Mills)	1 cup	111
SUGAR POPS or *SUGAR SMACKS* (Kellogg's)	1 cup	109
SUGAR SUBSTITUTE (Dia-Mel)	1 packet	3
*****SUKI-YAKI** (Durkee)	1 cup	293
SUNFLOWER SEED:		
Hulled (Planters)	1 oz.	164
Dry roasted (Flavor House)	1 oz.	178
SUNNY DOODLE (Drake's)	1 cake	141
SUZY Q (Hostess)	1 cake	268
SWEETBREADS, calf, braised	3 oz.	143
SWEET POTATO:		
Baked, peeled	5" x 2" sweet potato	155

Food and Description	Measure or Quantity	Calories
Canned, heavy syrup (Del Monte)	½ cup	138
Frozen:		
Candied (Mrs. Paul's)	⅓ pkg.	186
Candied yams (Birds Eye)	⅓ pkg.	215
*SWISS BURGER (Jeno's)	¼ of 30-oz. pkg.	374
SWISS ROLL (Drake's)	1 roll	376
SWISS STEAK:		
(Stouffer's)	10-oz. pkg.	569
(Swanson)	10-oz. dinner	361
SWORDFISH, broiled	3" x 3" x ½" steak	218

T

Food and Description	Measure or Quantity	Calories
TABASCO	¼ tsp.	<1
TACO:		
(Patio)	2¼-oz. taco	179
Cocktail (Patio)	½-oz. taco	39
TAMALE:		
Canned (Hormel)	1 tamale	80
Frozen (Banquet)	2 tamales with sauce	279
TANG, grape, grapefruit or orange	½ cup	61
TANGERINE (Sunkist)	1 large tangerine	39
*TANGERINE JUICE, frozen (Minute Maid, Snow Crop)	½ cup	57
TAPIOCA PUDDING:		
Chilled (Sealtest)	4 oz.	130
Canned (Hunt's)	5-oz. can	166
Mix, chocolate (Royal)	½ cup	186
TASTE AMERICA:		
New Orleans	⅓ pkg.	77
San Francisco	⅓ pkg.	35
TEA, instant		
* (Lipton)	1 cup	0
(Tender Leaf)	1 rounded tsp.	1
*Lemon flavored (Lipton)	1 cup	3
TEA, canned (Lipton)	8 fl. oz.	98

Food and Description	Measure or Quantity	Calories
TEAM, cereal	1⅓ cups	107
TEA, MIX, iced:		
Nestea	3 tsps.	58
Lemon flavored:		
*(Lipton)	1 cup	102
*Low calorie (Lipton)	1 cup	4
TEEM, soft drink	8 fl. oz.	122
TEMPTYS (Tastykake) butter creme, chocolate or lemon	⅔-oz. cake	94
TEXTURED VEGETABLE PROTEIN:		
Breakfast link, *Morningstar Farms*	1 link	54
Burger Builder (Betty Crocker)	¼ cup	60
Pathmark Plus	4 oz.	178
*Hamburger (Williams)	4 oz.	216
*Spaghetti sauce (Williams)	4 oz.	118
THUNDERBIRD WINE (Gallo):		
14% alcohol	1 fl. oz.	29
20% alcohol	1 fl. oz.	35
THURINGER (Oscar Mayer)	.8-oz. slice	74
TIA MARIA (Hiram Walker)	1½ fl. oz.	138
TOASTER CAKE:		
Corn Treats (Arnold)	1 piece	111
Toastee (Howard Johnson):		
Blueberry	1 piece	121
Cinnamon raisin	1 piece	114
Corn	1 piece	112
Pound	1 piece	111
Toaster Sandwich (Borden):		
Zesty or grilled cheese	1 sandwich	166
Pizza	1 sandwich	157
Toastette (Nabisco):		
Apple, blueberry, strawberry	1 piece	184
Brown sugar, cinnamon	1 piece	189
Cherry	1 piece	182
Orange marmalade	1 piece	181
Toast-r-Cake (Thomas'):		
Bran	1 piece	116
Corn	1 piece	118
Orange	1 piece	117
TOFFEE KRUNCH BAR (Sealtest)	3 fl. oz.	149
TOMATO:		
Cherry, whole	4 pieces	14

Food and Description	Measure or Quantity	Calories
Regular, whole	1 med.	33
Canned, sliced (Contadina)	½ cup	36
TOMATO JUICE:		
(Del Monte)	½ cup	22
(Heinz)	5½-fl.-oz. can	34
(Libby's)	½ cup	23
(Sacramento)	½ cup	24
TOMATO JUICE COCKTAIL:		
Snap-E-Tom	½ cup	24
Tomato Plus (Sacramento)	5½-fl.-oz. can	49
TOMATO SALAD, jellied (Contadina)	½ cup	60
TOMATO SOUP:		
Canned, regular pack:		
* (Campbell)	1 cup	79
* (Heinz) California	1 cup	81
(Heinz-*Great American*)	1 cup	168
*Canned, dietetic pack, with rice (Slim-ette)	8 oz.	34
Mix, cream of:		
(Lipton-*Cup-a-Soup*)	1 pkg.	98
(Wyler's)	1 pkg.	96
TOM COLLINS MIX:		
Canned (Party Tyme) 10% alcohol	3 fl. oz.	87
Mix, dry (Holland House)	1 serving	69
Mix, dry (Party Tyme)	½-oz. pkg.	50
Mix, liquid (Holland House)	2 fl. oz.	133
TOM COLLINS SOFT DRINK:		
(Canada Dry; Kirsch; Yukon Club)	8 fl. oz.	81
(Dr. Brown's; Hoffman; Shasta)	8 fl. oz.	85
TONGUE, beef, braised	3 oz.	208
TONGUE, canned (Hormel)	1 oz.	67
TOPPING:		
Butterscotch (Smucker's)	1 T.	66
Caramel, peanut butter (Smucker's)	1 T.	61
Chocolate, low calorie (Tillie Lewis)	1 T.	8
Chocolate fudge (Hershey's)	1 T.	54
Pecan in syrup (Smucker's)	1 T.	61
Pineapple (Kraft)	1 oz.	80
Spoonmallow (Kraft)	1 oz.	83
Walnut (Kraft)	1 oz.	113
TOPPING, WHIPPED:		
(Birds Eye) *Cool Whip*	1 T.	16

Food and Description	Measure or Quantity	Calories
(Lucky Whip)	1 T.	12
(Sealtest) *Zip Whip*	1 T.	8
TORTILLA	.7-oz. tortilla	42
TOTAL (General Mills)	1¼ cups	100
TRAMINER WINE (Inglenook)	1 fl. oz.	20
TRIPLE SEC LIQUEUR:		
(Bols)	1½ fl. oz.	152
(DeKuyper)	1½ fl. oz.	150
(Garnier)	1½ fl. oz.	124
TRIX, cereal (General Mills)	1 cup	110
TROPICAL PUNCH DRINK (Wagner)	8 fl. oz.	134
TUNA:		
Canned in oil:		
Solids & liq:		
Chunk (Star-Kist)	6½-oz. can	535
Solid (Star-Kist)	7-oz. can	577
Drained:		
Chunk, light (Chicken of the Sea)	6½-oz. can	294
((Bumble Bee)	1 cup	334
Canned in water (Chicken of the Sea)	7-oz. can	240
Canned, dietetic (Star-Kist)	6½-oz. can	207
TUNA PIE:		
(Banquet)	8-oz. pie	479
(Morton)	8-oz. pie	384
TUNA SALAD, home recipe	3 oz.	145
TURBOT, Greenland:		
Frozen (Weight Watchers)	18-oz. dinner	426
Frozen, with apple (Weight Watchers)	9½-oz. luncheon	277
TURKEY, roasted:		
Flesh & skin	3 oz.	190
Light meat	4" x 2" x ¼" slice	75
Dark meat	2½" x 1⅝" x ¼" slice	43
TURKEY DINNER:		
(Banquet)	11-oz. dinner	293
(Morton) sliced	11-oz. dinner	346
(Morton) 3-course	16¾-oz. dinner	613
(Swanson) 3-course	16-oz. dinner	501
(Weight Watchers)	18-oz. dinner	302

Food and Description	Measure or Quantity	Calories
TURKEY PIE:		
(Banquet)	8-oz. pie	415
(Swanson)	8-oz. pie	422
TURKEY SOUP MIX, noodle		
(Lipton)	½ cup	30
TURKEY TETRAZZINI (Morton)	11-oz. dinner	396
TWINKIE (Hostess) chocolate	1 cake	162

V

Food and Description	Measure or Quantity	Calories
VALPOLICELLA WINE (Antinori)	1 fl. oz.	28
VANDERMINT	1½-fl. oz.	135
VANILLA EXTRACT		
(Virginia Dare)	1 tsp.	10
VANILLA ICE CREAM:		
(Borden) 10.5% fat	¼ pt.	132
Lady Borden 14% fat	¼ pt.	162
(Meadow Gold) 10% fat	¼ pt.	126
(Sealtest-*Party Slice*)	¼ pt.	133
(Sealtest) 10.2% fat	¼ pt.	133
(Sealtest) 12.1% fat	¼ pt.	144
French (Prestige)	¼ pt.	183
Fudge royale (Sealtest)	¼ pt.	132
VANILLA ICE MILK		
(Borden-*Lite Line*)	¼ pt.	108
VANILLA PUDDING:		
(Del Monte)	5-oz. container	190
(Hunt's)	5-oz. container	238
(Royal-*Creamerino*)	5-oz. container	217
Chilled (Breakstone)	5-oz. container	252
*Mix (Royal)	½ cup	163
VEAL, broiled, medium-cooked:		
Loin, chop	3 oz.	199
Steak or cutlet, lean & fat	3 oz.	184
Roasted, rib	3 oz.	229
VEAL DINNER:		
Parmigiana (Banquet)	11-oz. dinner	421
Parmigiana (Swanson)	12¼-oz. dinner	492
Parmigiana (Weight Watchers)	9½-oz. luncheon	260
Breaded veal with spaghetti in tomato sauce (Swanson)	8¼-oz. pkg.	272
V-8 (Campbell)	½ cup	21

Food and Description	Measure or Quantity	Calories
VEGETABLES, mixed:		
Canned (Veg-All)	½ cup	39
(Birds Eye)	½ cup	50
Chinese (Birds Eye)	⅓ pkg.	65
Chinese (La Choy)	½ cup	11
In butter sauce (Green Giant)	⅓ pkg.	67
VEGETABLE SOUP:		
Canned, regular pack:		
* (Campbell) old fashioned	1 cup	70
*Beef (Heinz)	1 cup	66
With beef broth (Heinz-*Great American*)	1 cup	144
Vegetarian:		
* (Campbell)	1 cup	71
* (Heinz)	1 cup	83
*Canned, dietetic pack (Slim-ette)	8 oz.	46
*Mix, beef (Lipton)	1 cup	58
VERMOUTH:		
Dry & extra dry:		
(Lejon; Noilly Pratt)	1 fl. oz.	33
(Tribuno)	1 fl. oz.	30
Sweet:		
(Lejon; Tribuno)	1 fl. oz.	45
(Noilly Pratt)	1 fl. oz.	43
VERNORS:		
Regular	8 fl. oz.	93
Low calorie	8 fl. oz.	1
VICHYSSOISE SOUP (Crosse & Blackwell)	½ of 13-oz. can	94
VIENNA SAUSAGE:		
(Armour Star)	.6-oz. sausage	45
(Van Camp)	1 oz.	68
VINEGAR	1 T.	2
VIN KAFE (Lejon)	1 fl. oz.	61
VIRGIN SOUR MIX (Party Tyme)	½-oz. pkg.	50
VODKA SCREWDRIVER (Old Mr. Boston) 25 proof	3 fl. oz.	117

W

WAFFLE, buttermilk, frozen (Aunt Jemima)	1 section	57

Food and Description	Measure or Quantity	Calories
WALNUT, English or Persian (Diamond)	6 halves	40
WATERCRESS	½ cup	3
WATERMELON:		
Wedge	4" x 8" wedge	111
Diced	½ cup	21
WELSH RAREBIT, canned (Snow)	4 oz.	171
WHEAT CHEX (Ralston Purina)	⅔ cup	115
WHEAT GERM CEREAL:		
Cinnamon raisin (Kretschmer)	¼ cup	110
Plain (Pillsbury)	¼ cup	120
*WHEATENA	½ cup	88
WHEATIES	1¼ cups	101
*WHIP 'N CHILL (Jell-O):		
All flavors except chocolate	½ cup	135
Chocolate	½ cup	144
WHISKEY SOUR:		
(Hiram Walker)	3 fl. oz.	177
(National Distillers-*Duet*) 12½% alcohol	8-fl.-oz. can	256
Dry mix (Bar-Tender's)	1 serving	79
Dry mix (Holland House)	1 serving	69
Dry mix (Party Tyme)	½-oz. pkg.	50
Liquid mix (Holland House)	2 fl. oz.	109
WHITEFISH, LAKE:		
Baked, stuffed	3 oz.	183
Smoked	3 oz.	132
WILD RICE (Gourmet House)	⅛ cup	75
WINE Petri) Vino Rosso or Bianco	1 fl. oz.	22
WINK (Canada Dry)	8 fl. oz.	113
WON TON SOUP (Mow Sang)	10-oz. can	67

Y

YANKEE DOODLES (Drake's)	1-oz. cake	120
YODEL (Drake's)	1 roll	116

Food and Description	Measure or Quantity	Calories
YOGURT:		
Plain:		
(Dean)	8-oz. container	143
(Dannon)	8-oz. container	136
Apple, Dutch (Axelrod)	8-oz. container	228
Apricot:		
(Breakstone)	8-oz. container	220
(Breakstone-*Swiss Parfait*)	8-oz. container	249
(Dannon)	8-oz. container	258
Blueberry:		
(Axelrod)	8-oz. container	226
(Breakstone)	8-oz. container	252
(Breakstone-*Swiss Parfait*)	8-oz. container	296
(Dannon)	8-oz. container	258
(Dean)	8-oz. container	259
(Meadow Gold)	8-oz. container	249
(Sealtest-*Light n' Lively*)	8-oz. container	257
(SugarLo)	8-oz. container	117
Boysenberry:		
(Dannon)	8-oz. container	258
(Meadow Gold)	8-oz. container	249
Cherry:		
(Dannon)	8-oz. container	258
(Dean)	8-oz. container	245
Black (SugarLo)	8-oz. container	117
Coffee (Dannon)	8-oz. container	198
Danny (Dannon):		
Cuplet, any flavor	4-oz. container	129
Frozen pop	2½-oz. pop	127
Lemon:		
(Breakstone-*Swiss Parfait*)	8-oz. container	254
(Dannon)	8-oz. container	198
(Sealtest-*Light n' Lively*)	8-oz. container	229
Mandarin orange:		
(Borden) Swiss style	8-oz. container	227
(Breakstone-*Swiss Parfait*)	8-oz. container	263
Orange (Dean)	8-oz. container	311
Peach:		
(Axelrod)	8-oz. container	220
(Borden) Swiss style	8-oz. container	221
(Breakstone-*Swiss Parfait*)	8-oz. container	254
(Dean)	8-oz. container	259
(Sealtest-*Light n' Lively*)	8-oz. container	252
(SugarLo)	8-oz. container	118
Pineapple:		
(Dean)	8-oz. container	265
(Meadow Gold)	8-oz. container	249
(Sealtest-*Light n' Lively*)	8-oz. container	241
(SugarLo)	8-oz. container	118
Pineapple-cherry (Axelrod)	8-oz. container	229
Prune whip (Dannon)	8-oz. container	258

Food and Description	Measure or Quantity	Calories
Raspberry:		
(Axelrod)	8-oz. container	227
(Borden) Swiss style	8-oz. container	236
(Breakstone)	8-oz. container	249
(Dannon)	8-oz. container	258
(Dean)	8-oz. container	272
(Meadow Gold) Swiss style	8-oz. container	245
Red (Sealtest-*Light n' Lively*)	8-oz. container	225
(SugarLo)	8-oz. container	118
Strawberry:		
(Axelrod)	8-oz. container	224
(Borden) Swiss style	8-oz. container	227
(Breakstone)	8-oz. container	225
(Dannon)	8-oz. container	258
(Dean)	8-oz. container	256
(Meadow Gold)	8-oz. container	249
(Meadow Gold) Swiss style	8-oz. container	245
(Sealtest-*Light n' Lively*)	8-oz. container	234
(SugarLo)	8-oz. container	111
Vanilla:		
(Borden) Swiss style	8-oz. container	235
(Breakstone)	8-oz. container	195
(Dannon)	8-oz. container	198

Z

ZINFANDEL WINE (Inglenook)	1 fl. oz.	19
ZWIEBACK (Nabisco)	1 piece	31

More SIGNET and PLUME Books of Special Interest

☐ **JOGGING, AEROBICS AND DIET: One Is Not Enough—You Need All Three** by Roy Ald with a Foreword by M. Thomas Woodall, Ph.D. A personalized prescription for health, vitality and general well-being based on a revolutionary new theory of exercise. (#Y5540—$1.25)

☐ **THE SUPERMARKET HANDBOOK Access to Whole Foods** by Nikki and David Goldbeck. This book will prove invaluable to any shopper concerned with the quality and nutritive value of the foods available in today's supermarkets. It will help you to understand labels and select foods with a discerning eye, and provides easy, low-cost ways of preparing whole foods and using them to replace processed ones. "An enormously useful and heartening work!"—The New York Times (#Z5089—$3.95)

☐ **SECRETS FOR STAYING SLIM** by Lelord Kordel. Diet Naturally! A famous nutritionist and author of EAT AND GROW YOUNGER offers an organically correct guide to quick weight loss that keeps you trim and healthy. (#Y5128—$1.25)

☐ **YOGA FOR AMERICANS** by Indra Devi. A complete six-week home course in the widely recognized science that offers its practitioners a vital and confident approach to the pressures and tensions of modern living. (#Y4606—$1.25)

☐ **THE NEW AMERICAN MEDICAL DICTIONARY AND HEALTH MANUAL (revised)** by Robert Rothenberg, M.D. Over 8500 definitions of medical terms, disorders, and diseases, with more than 300 illustrations, make this the most complete and easy-to-understand book of its kind. Also includes a comprehensive first-aid section and guides to better health. (#J6284—$1.95)

THE NEW AMERICAN LIBRARY, INC.,
P.O. Box 999, Bergenfield, New Jersey 07621

Please send me the SIGNET and PLUME BOOKS I have checked above. I am enclosing $_____(check or money order—no currency or C.O.D.'s). Please include the list price plus 25¢ a copy to cover handling and mailing costs. (Prices and numbers are subject to change without notice.)

Name_____

Address_____

City_____State_____Zip Code_____
Allow at least 3 weeks for delivery